THE NEW baby book

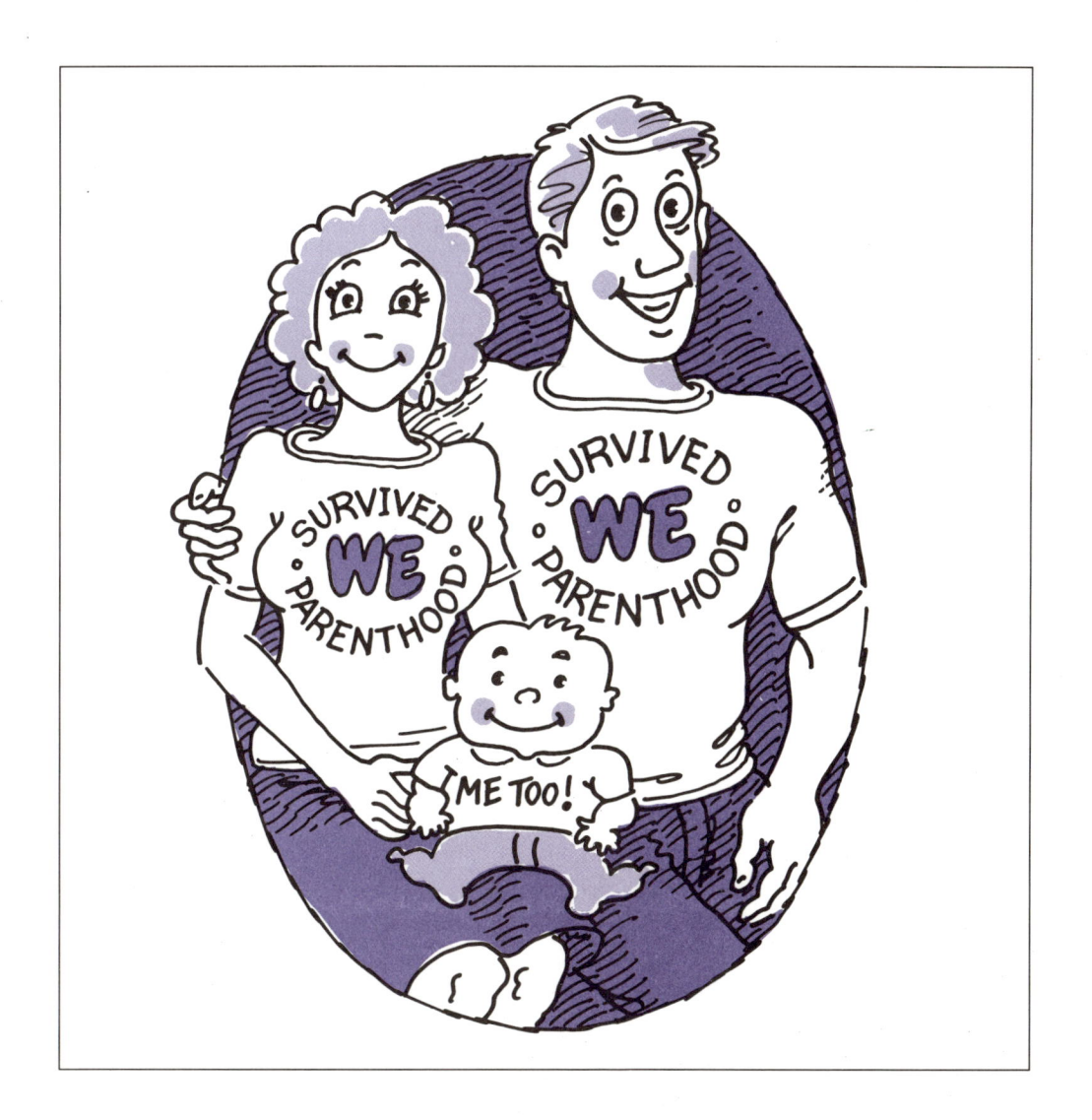

By Dr Howard W. Chilton
M.B., B.S., (Lond.), M.R.C.P. (UK), D.C.H. (Lond.)

*This book is dedicated to the girls in my life –
Tamara, Georgina and Isabella*

Illustrated by Tony Vuletich

CONTENTS

3 Introduction

4 Birth and Beyond

14 The Circumcision Decision

17 The Seal of Approval

28 Early Days

40 Breast Is Best

52 The New Baby Game

54 Settling In

57 Developmental Timetable

70 Colic And The Crying Baby

74 Losing A Little, Losing It All

77 Conclusion

78 Glossary

79 Index

EDITORIAL
Managing Editor: Judy Poulos
Editorial Co-ordinator: Margaret Kelly
UK Consultants: Helen Travis, Lyn Murray
Editorial Assistant: Ella Martin
Medical Editor: Jutta Sieverding
Index: Michael Wyatt

DESIGN AND PRODUCTION
Margie Mulray
Chris Hatcher
Cover Design: Frank Pithers

PHOTOGRAPHY
Front Cover: Jon Waddy, Styling: Sally Hirst
Back Cover: Andrew Elton

DESIGN AND PRODUCTION MANAGER
Nadia Sbisa

PUBLISHER
Philippa Sandall

The New Baby Book
ISBN 1 86343 071 7
Formatted by J.B. Fairfax Press Pty Ltd
Output by Adtype, Sydney
Printed by Toppan Printing Co, Hong Kong
Distributed by J.B. Fairfax Ltd
9 Trinity Centre, Park Farm Estate,
Wellingborough, Northants.
Ph: (0933) 402330 Fax: (0933) 402234

Family Circle is a registered trademark of IPC Magazines Ltd.
Published by J. B. Fairfax Press Pty Ltd by arrangement with IPC Magazines Ltd

© J. B. Fairfax Press Pty Ltd, 1990
This book is copyright. Apart from any fair dealing for the purpose of private study, research, criticism or review, as permitted under the Copyright Act, no part may be reproduced by any process without the written permission of the publisher. Enquiries should be made in writing to the publisher.

INTRODUCTION

This book was written to be a guide for new mothers during their first three months with their new baby. It is a time for looking after the baby and trying to catch up on sleep, not for reading, so the book is brief. After looking after mothers and their babies for over fifteen years, the last ten spent as Director of Newborn Care at the Royal Hospital for Women in Sydney, I have some idea of the questions that plague the new mother following birth, and of the incredible variety of answers that she'll be subjected to, some right, some wrong, and some laughable.

This book has some of the best answers I know. If it's not enough, add a lot of commonsense and a little trial and error.

It came as no surprise to those of us in the baby business, that it was the babies who survived the recent Mexican earthquake, not, alas, their mothers. Babies are as tough as old boots with an amazing ability to survive adverse conditions. They also come equipped with the ability to teach their mothers all they need to know about bringing up babies. In order for mum to tune into her little teacher, however, she must not fear making mistakes.

The only important error a mother can make is to seek answers from outside her relationship with her baby. That's when the trouble starts.

The reason isn't too subtle. Who doesn't find kittens cuddly? Even dog-haters like puppies and so it is with babies. Human infants are magnetically attractive to most people and give satisfaction out of proportion to their size. This was a very useful mechanism in the days when many mothers did not survive childbirth and someone in the vicinity had to care enough to take over the baby. Now that good antenatal care and obstetrics have virtually eliminated the danger to mother, the problem remains: everyone wants to get in on the act.

Everyone wants to 'help' mother – that is, to persuade her to do it **their** way. Babies are so adaptable that virtually any way, as long as it's half reasonable, will work. So there are about fifty thousand ways to bring up a baby and they are all successful.

New mothers do sometimes feel in need of advice, particularly if they are having problems, with breastfeeding for example. Don't seek advice from all and sundry – find someone you trust and listen only to them. Conflicting advice is one of the greatest problems new mothers have. Be wary of advice. If it does not sound sensible, if it implies that babies are fragile objects that will break like eggshells unless handled in a particular way, if it suggests you need a degree in dietetics, paediatrics, hygiene and psychology to really understand – **then ignore it!** Humanity is no worse off than the rest of the animal kingdom and nature has endowed all mothers with an instinctive knowledge of how to look after their baby. This knowledge does not lie in the intellect, or in books – not even this one. It lies in the heart, the instinct and in the soft inner voice that says 'try this' or 'that advice doesn't sound right, I'll try this instead'. If you feel he's hungry, feed him. If he's not, he'll tell you and the next time he cries like that, you will know.

Don't get bogged down in the 'right way' – there isn't one! There's just you and your baby, a unique combination, doing it together for the first time.

During the course of this book I will always refer to mother as 'she' (I'm sure no-one will object) and to the baby as 'he' (some might). I am not sexist and I love girl babies too (I have two at home) but it's much less confusing than the 'he/she' alternative.

BIRTH AND BEYOND

All the months of waiting are finally over. You've been to the ante-natal classes, painted furniture, shopped for baby clothes and made endless plans. You have dreamed about the birth of your baby, and no doubt worried about how it would go, and then after what seems like an eternity the day finally arrives!

Don't set your standards too high

EXPECTATIONS

I once had a 'celebrity patient' whose baby got into minor trouble at birth by inhaling a bit of meconium. He puffed and panted and needed a bit of oxygen for a few hours. He remained in the special care nursery for three days and then joined his mother in the post-natal ward. Things did not go smoothly there either. There were feeding difficulties, sticky eyes, phototherapy for jaundice, a depressed mum ... the works! Eventually everything sorted itself out and mother and baby went home in good shape.

Imagine the position of my eyebrows when, a couple of months later, I picked up a women's magazine of enormous circulation to see a feature on this lady's experience of childbirth. She was evidently Mother Earth herself, from the spiritual delivery to the gentle lying-in, from the smooth breastfeeding regimen to the ideal baby at home. All was easy, fulfilling, natural and suffused with a warm, pink glow...

What a missed opportunity! If only she had told her vast readership the way it *really* was! How much more good it would have done. If only she had told of the agony as well as the ecstasy, instead of yet another impossibly ideal story. Yet another role model out of Hollywood that we have come to expect as normal.

Not surprisingly, therefore, some mothers go through pregnancy and into delivery with their expectations just a little too high. They are expecting a quick, painless, ideal delivery, producing a perfect, beautiful, responsive infant who then breastfeeds like a natural. This does occur and if it does you're very lucky.

Alas, in reality things are usually not quite as picturesque. Contractions are a good deal more painful than many mothers expect although some mothers are just lucky and have an easier time than others. Not only do pain thresholds vary greatly but so does the actual power of the contractions. Do not allow someone else to tell you how much pain you ought to be able to cope with. There is no pain easier to bear than somebody else's! Feeling guilty about the need for analgesia is too common in labour wards and birth centres and is so unnecessary. Labour should not be more painful than you can stand and

BIRTH AND BEYOND

your baby can only benefit if you are comfortable enough to relax and enjoy the experience.

Some babies also decide that labour is too hard and insist upon being delivered by Caesarean section. In fact, this is up to fifteen per cent of births in some urban populations. So you should accept in advance the idea that it might be necessary for you and your baby.

Following birth many babies prefer to spend the first day or so sleeping and are reluctant to feed. He may virtually ignore his mother who has worked so hard to bring him into the world. Don't take it personally, just accept that labour and its aftermath may not be ideal and don't set too high a standard for yourself or your baby.

THE FIRST BREATH

How the system works
Within the womb the fetus floats in his ocean of amniotic fluid, supplied with oxygen and food from his mother's circulation through the placenta. His circulation bypasses the lungs through a couple of channels, one (called the foramen ovale or oval window) within the heart and the other (called the ductus arteriosus or arterial channel) outside. His lungs are filled with fluid and although he makes shallow breathing movements, his lungs are not used for absorbing oxygen.

On delivery many changes have to be made to adapt to living independently on dry land. The baby needs to get rid of about half a cupful (125 mL) of fluid from his lungs and this he does – usually rapidly. A third of it is squeezed out into his mouth when his chest is compressed by the birth canal (in a vaginal birth) and the rest is absorbed into his circulation following the first breath. In a Caesarean delivery, all the fluid must be absorbed by his circulation. At the same time, under the combined stimulus of light, the cool air on his cheek, the different noise level and a rise in blood-oxygen caused by his first breath, his circulation undergoes radical change.

With the first breath the channels which bypass the lungs constrict and close and the blood vessels in the lungs open up. This forces the blood through the lungs on each

On delivery your baby has to make many changes to adapt to living independently

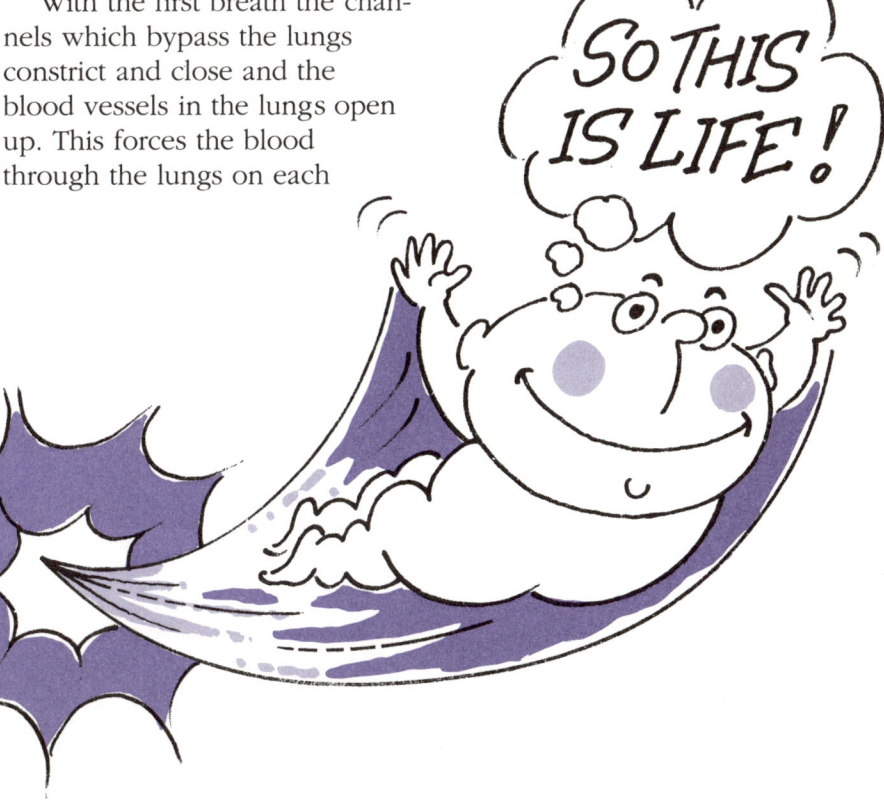

BIRTH AND BEYOND

Babies are perfectly designed for delivery

circulation, where it absorbs oxygen from the air waiting in the lungs from the breath. This oxygen is then carried to the body. Normally, this process is rapid and smooth and no help is required at the birth.

SLOW TO START

Some babies terrify their parents by taking their own good time to start breathing after birth and these babies may be grateful for a little assistance. A little gentle suctioning of the mouth and throat, usually to remove mucus, blood, or fluid from the lung sometimes provides an extra stimulus to the breathing drive. If this is not enough the lungs can be inflated using a tight-fitting rubber mask and a venti-lator bag. Following this, most of the babies who require help will be stimulated to continue breathing on their own. Now and again, especially if the babies are sick or the lungs are not mature, more resuscitation is required. A tube the size of a drinking straw may be inserted into the baby's windpipe ('intu-bation') and the lungs inflated directly with the ventilation bag.

It is helpful to appreciate how well designed babies are for delivery and how long they can manage without oxygen before any permanent harm ensues. A baby has to be totally without oxygen for at least twenty minutes before the brain can come to any permanent harm. Should the drive to start breathing on delivery be suppressed, the baby will be given help to get things going long before this occurs.

If your baby has been stretched beyond his ability to compensate, your paediatrician will be able to detect it within the first twelve to twenty-four hours. If your baby remains well during this time he has clearly coped with the situation.

MECONIUM STAINING

There is one group of babies which is given special attention at delivery. In about ten per cent of births, the amniotic fluid is stained with meconium (fetal stool). Meconium is a thick, treacly substance that is harm-less as long as it doesn't get deep into the baby's lungs. If it does, it acts as an irritant to the lining of the air passages and generally gums up the works. This can cause pneumonia and other lung problems.

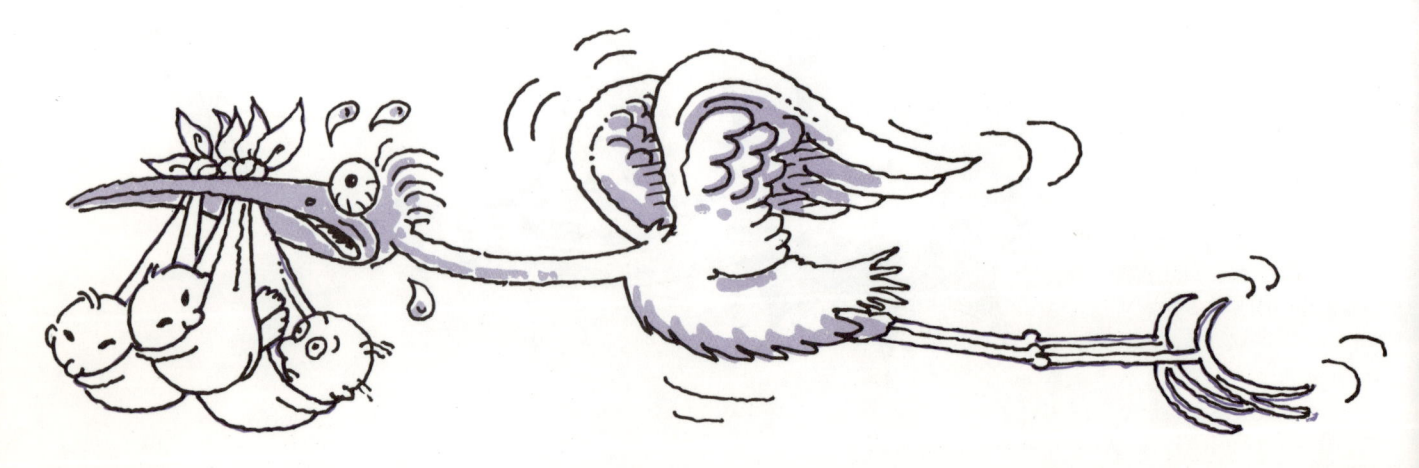

BIRTH AND BEYOND

Consequently, when this baby's head emerges, his throat and nose are sucked out to remove any trace of meconium before he has had a chance to breathe. This will prevent him from inhaling it. If this meconium is difficult to remove he may be intubated at delivery to make sure that there is no meconium down his airway. This is good preventative medicine and will do him no harm.

VITAMIN K

Soon after your baby is born, he will be offered an injection of vitamin K. This practice is pretty universal, and for good reason.

Until thirty years ago there was an important, common and lethal condition of babies called 'haemorrhagic disease of the newborn'. Typically a few days after delivery, the baby's clotting system would cease to work efficiently, and bleeding, often severe, would occur from the umbilical cord or the bowel. He would often recover spontaneously if the haemorrhage was minor but if it was brisk he could rapidly develop shock caused by the loss of blood and unless treated could die. The treatment was transfusion and vitamin K.

What does vitamin K do?
The blood-clotting system of the body is based on a complex series of reactions between many proteins and chemicals called clotting factors. Many of these require vitamin K for their activation and without it, poor coagulation results. When this was realised, the use of a routine injection of vitamin K after birth became commonplace and the disease virtually disappeared.

That is until the last ten years or so. Since then there has been a growing number of reports of haemorrhagic disease. However, it seems to have taken a new, and deadly, form. It may not be present in the first week but four to six weeks after delivery. More seriously, the bleeding is often in the brain. The babies in these recent reports have two things in common. Firstly, they did not receive an injection of vitamin K after birth and, secondly, they were all exclusively breastfed. Studies have shown that most healthy babies born at full-term are not born short of vitamin K. However, by the third day of life, as they start to grow, so vitamin K deficiency can emerge. Giving vitamin K to the mother before delivery does not seem to help as it passes across the placenta only poorly. Anyway, many mothers have relatively low levels of vitamin K in their blood towards the end of their pregnancy.

We also know that breast milk contains only very small amounts of vitamin K. Cow's milk and commercial infant formula appear to contain very much higher levels than breast milk (up to ten times as much). However, if a nursing mother is supplied with adequate vitamin K in her diet, a little will appear in her milk and be absorbed by the baby. So if you are breastfeeding it is a good idea to eat fresh, leafy vegetables every day as this is a rich source of this important vitamin.

Why has this disease reappeared?
There are probably two reasons.

Vitamin K is vital, and it's completely safe. Don't let your baby miss out on this injection

BIRTH AND BEYOND

Fresh, leafy vegetables are a rich source of vitamin K

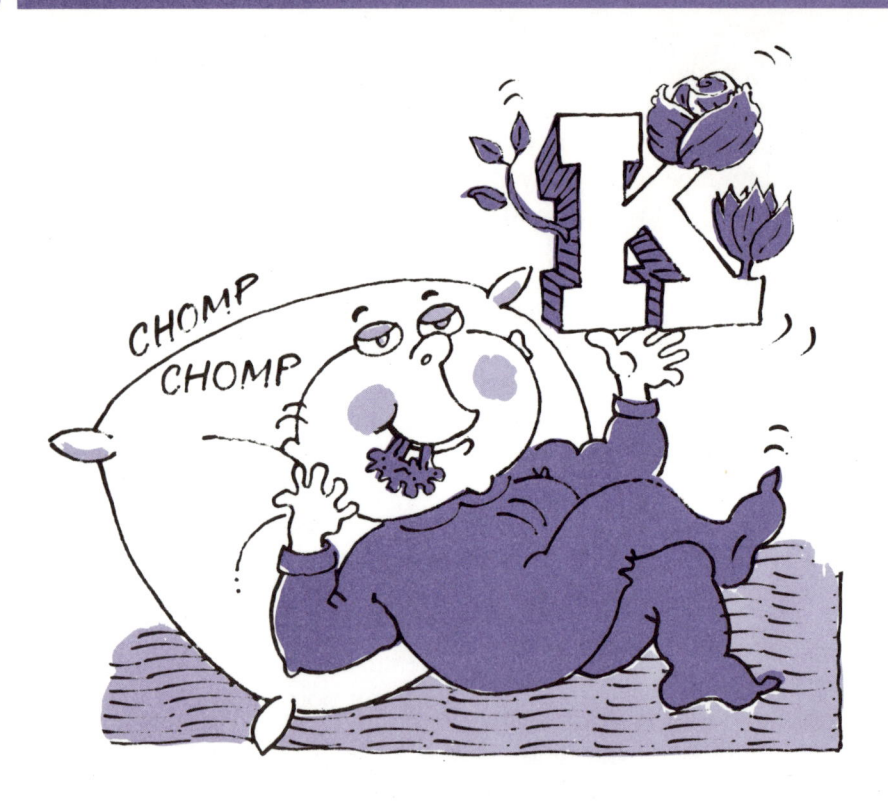

Firstly, with the recent movement against technology in birthing there are some babies whose parents refuse the vitamin K injection offered to every newborn baby.

Secondly, a few years ago most babies received at least a little formula or cow's milk as supplement, even when fully breastfed, and this small amount was enough to boost the baby's vitamin K level and avoid deficiency. Nowadays, largely misplaced anxiety about cow's milk allergy means it is more likely that he will receive no such supplement.

The injection of vitamin K
The preparation of vitamin K used nowadays is completely safe. It is a synthetic version of the natural vitamin and never causes a problem. It is best given by intramuscular injection as we can guarantee full absorption. A single injection is enough for the baby's needs until he is eating his own vegetables and absorbing his own vitamin K.

It is also likely that vitamin K is absorbed when given to the baby by mouth. Unfortunately, many babies vomit mucus in the first hours and it is difficult to know how much is absorbed. If the vitamin is given in this way the baby should be given double the injected dose. This is a good idea for the babies whose parents adamantly refuse the injection.

POSTNATAL CONTRACTIONS

You may find that every time you breastfeed your baby you develop quite painful contractions of the womb. These pains also seem to be more uncomfortable (that is maternity hospital jargon for 'painful') as you have more pregnancies. These problem contractions tend to disappear in the first few days.

BIRTH AND BEYOND

A lot has been said and written about bonding over the last several years which seems to imply that it is a straightforward mechanism. This approach says that if you don't see and hold your baby immediately on delivery, always have him in sight and breastfeed him, then your relationship may never recover!

BONDING

This black and white approach may be appropriate for lower animals like rats, sheep and goats but for such a complex organism as a human being it is manifestly untrue. Not only does it defy commonsense (and what we all know about adopting parents), but careful scientific studies have shown that our system is far more complex than this. Humans possess great flexibility and enormous ability to cope with adverse circumstances at birth and after.

However, that is not to say that it's *all* rubbish. If the mother has a comfortable delivery, comes from a stable family, is conscious during her baby's birth, the delivery lives up to her expectations and is not too painful, she breastfeeds the baby early and has him in her room with her in the postnatal period, this mother will probably have an *easier* time falling in love with her baby and feeling confident about meeting his needs after she goes home.

If she misses any of those factors it will make either none, or very little, difference to her abilities *in the end* but it is possible she could have more difficulty getting to feel comfortable with her baby. By 'difficulty' it doesn't mean she has to try harder but that the instincts to look after her baby may flow less easily and the process may take a little longer.

It is also unrewarding to compare, as some experts have, the bonding behaviour of, say sheep, with humans and try to derive reasonable conclusions that apply to human mothers and their babies. For instance, a mother ewe bonds instantly with

Getting to love your baby is not always easy

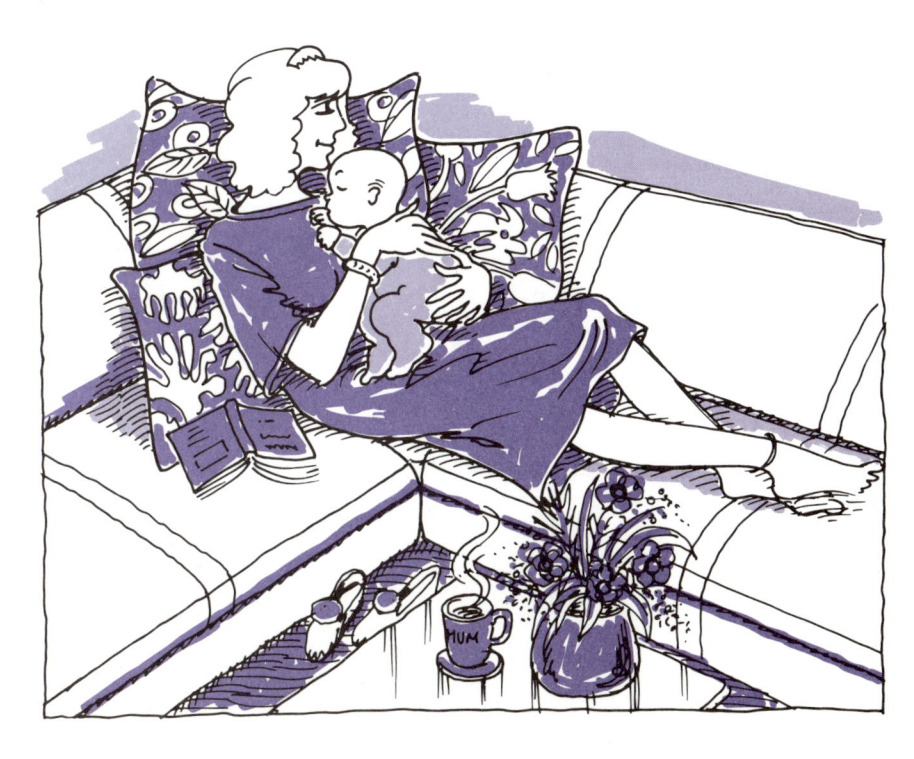

BIRTH AND BEYOND

Bonding is the right word – you're stuck for life

her newborn lamb at birth and that bond can easily be disrupted if it is not allowed to occur straight after delivery.

Why should biology arrange one system for sheep and another for humans? Sheep all deliver their lambs at the same time. Imagine three hundred ewes and three hundred lambs all milling around in a field. If ewe and lamb did not immediately attach to each other there could be a lot of confusion in that paddock at feed-time.

Humans in prehistoric times lived in small groups of perhaps ten or fifteen in number. There would only be two or three babies at the most in any group and they would have been delivered at different times. This would give the mothers ample opportunity to get to know their own baby – and the babies would also be shared to some degree with the other women in the group.

Leboyer – fact or fad?
The great fashion for Leboyer deliveries was based upon the belief that a quiet, non-clinical atmosphere is preferable at the delivery, which is true, and that the baby's relationship with his parents, his behaviour and security would be improved in the long term, which is not true. It has been demonstrated in carefully controlled studies that, after one year, there is no

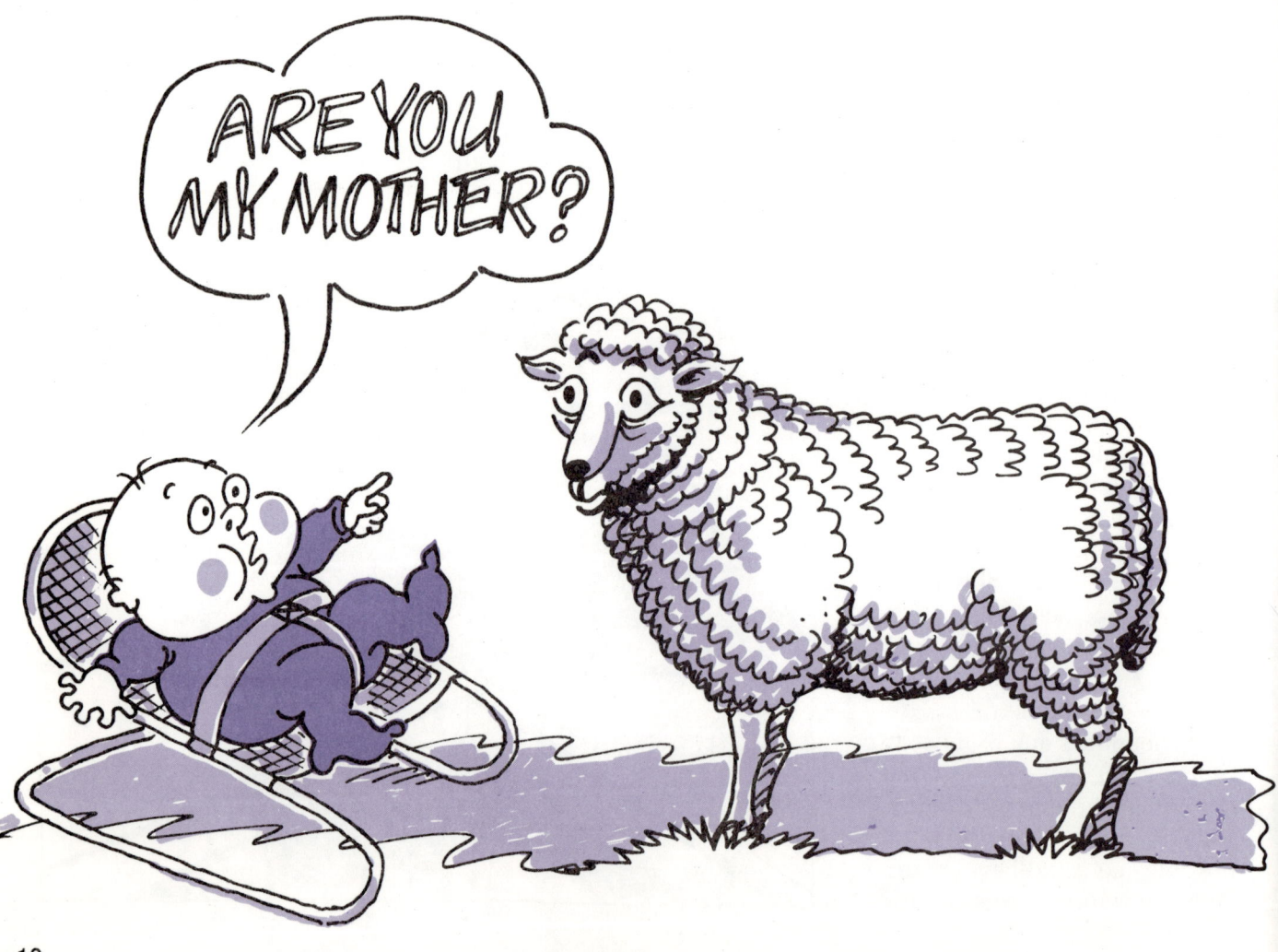

BIRTH AND BEYOND

discernible difference in the babies born of Leboyer deliveries compared to babies born of routine deliveries.

So don't misunderstand me. Factors which enhance bonding are excellent and should be encouraged because they make the task of getting to love your baby easier. But if you miss any of them because, for instance, you have a general anaesthetic for a Caesarean section, or your baby has to spend twenty-four hours in the special care unit, or you decide to bottle-feed for whatever reason, don't worry – your bond will be just as strong, and 'bond' is the right word – you're stuck for life!

IT TAKES TIME TO FALL IN LOVE WITH YOUR BABY

This message was on a banner draped across the nursery in the hospital of the famous English paediatrician, Sir Hugh Jolly. He recognised how many mothers worried that there they were five days after the birth and the baby was still "just a baby". No pink glow, no rending hearts, he's just a blob – and a noisy one at that. If you feel like that about your baby, be reassured that many other mothers feel just the same – and *they* hate to admit the way they feel too.

A study showed that over thirty per cent of mothers still felt indifferent about their babies after several days, and some mothers took over a month before they felt comfortable with their baby. We are all different. We all deal with changes and accept new people into our lives at a different pace and in different ways. Give it at least three months before you start to worry. And then if you still can't stand him because he looks like your mother-in-law, perhaps you had better talk it over with your doctor who will put you in touch with people who can help you.

RESPONSIVENESS

'When will my baby be able to see?'

It is sad that many parents don't realise how incredibly responsive their baby is to things around him in the first few days and weeks after birth.

First and foremost, don't believe those people who tell you babies can't see for weeks. They see *clearly*. They are, however, a little short-sighted focusing best at a distance of about twenty centimetres (eight inches). Not only do they see well but, within just a few minutes of delivery, babies will often show a 'face-searching' reflex. Babies actually have a preference for looking at the human face over other patterns or objects. Many will stare at mother or father for long periods in the early hours after birth – a sure-fire way to melt a heart. The baby also learns to recognise his mother's smell within a few days of birth and has definite taste preference. He certainly responds positively to touch, enjoying stroking and relishing skin-to-skin contact.

Most fascinating is the fact that he has the ability to imitate a facial expression shown to him. Get him in a quiet, alert mood and try sticking out your

Many parents don't realise how incredibly responsive their baby is to things around him during the first few days and weeks

BIRTH AND BEYOND

You can usually recognise a new father; he's the one with terminal fatigue in his smiling muscles

tongue to him. Within just a few days of birth he will try to stick out his tongue too.

And to think that it wasn't so long ago that people thought babies were just blobs for the first few weeks! Far from it – your baby is a real person right from day one.

FROM HUSBAND TO FATHER

It cannot be a coincidence that so many diverse cultures exclude fathers from the birth process. It is as if they fear that father might get too involved in his newborn baby and neglect his role as provider. It just would not do for dad to spend all day playing with his baby by the hearth when there is no food in the pantry. Studies of fathers' response to their newborns seem to validate this conclusion. If they were very involved in the birth process, most fathers exhibit much the same behaviour as mothers when presented with their babies – some taking quite a dominant role in handling and playing with the baby. Certainly, they seemed totally engrossed with the little one and positively bursting with self-esteem. You can usually recognise a new dad; he's the one with terminal fatigue in his smiling muscles.

It must be said that a father cannot be as involved with his baby as a breastfeeding mother. Babies tend to treat their fathers

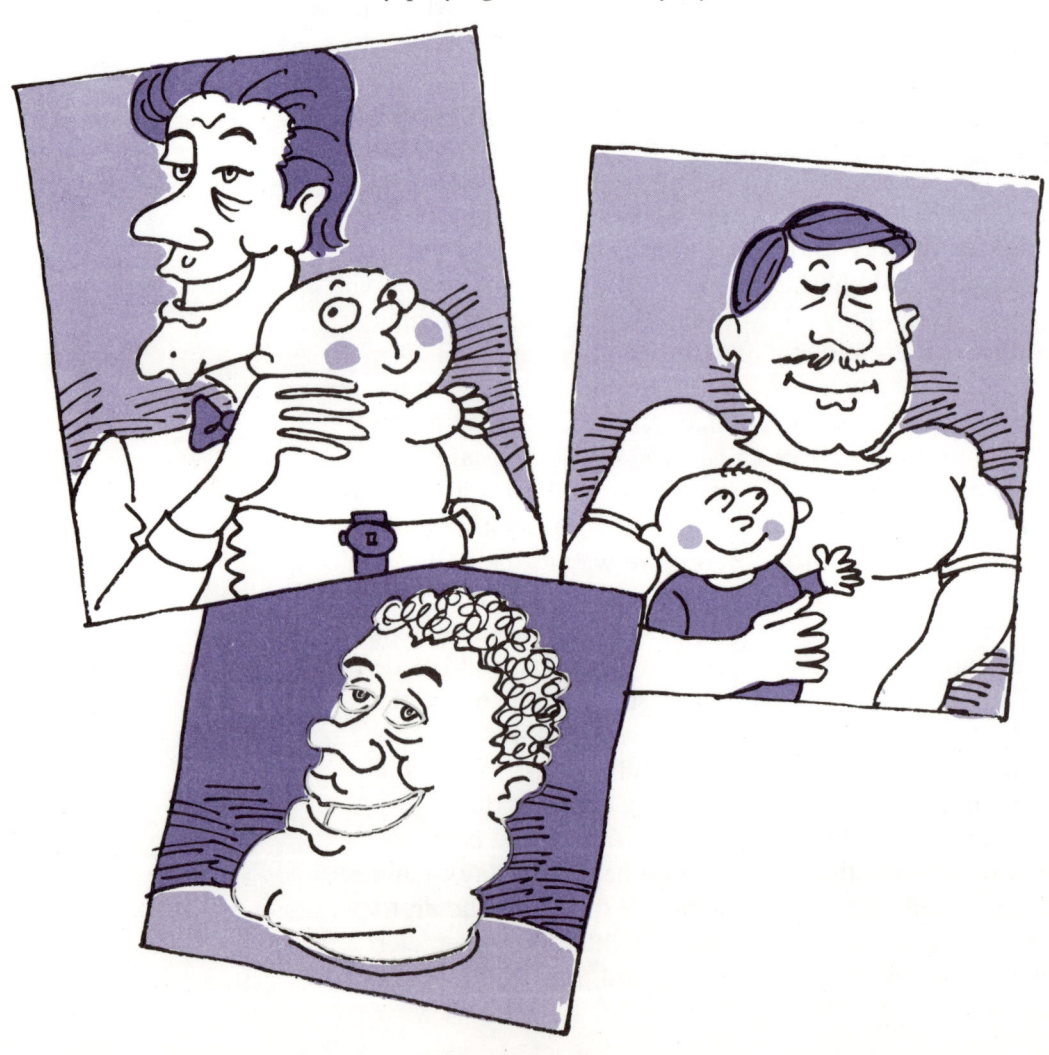

BIRTH AND BEYOND

with indifference for a few weeks, as they are mostly interested in the smell, taste and milk of their mother. Most fathers can handle this without getting upset or jealous but it is a good idea to involve father as much as possible in all of the care-taking activities he can do. Literally, the more he does for the baby, the closer he will feel to him. This is one of the small advantages of bottle-feeding, allowing the parenting role to be divided more equally between mother and father.

Superdad
Some early studies on bonding assessed the closeness of the relationship between mother and baby, using a description of the way mother behaved while the doctor examined her baby. If she stood on the other side of the room, gazing out of the window and when the baby cried, turned around and muttered, 'Oh, he's always doing that', she scored a big zero. If she stood next to the doctor and immediately pacified him when he cried (the baby, that is – doctors are pretty brave), she scored a six.

I recently had a big burly dockside worker and his wife in my consulting room, for their baby's check-up. Mother had been quite sick and had to remain in hospital for four weeks following the birth of her baby. Hence her husband had looked after all the baby's needs and had bottle-fed him. When I examined the baby, I had to contend with an enormous shoulder in my way, as father got a score of seven out of six for bonding!

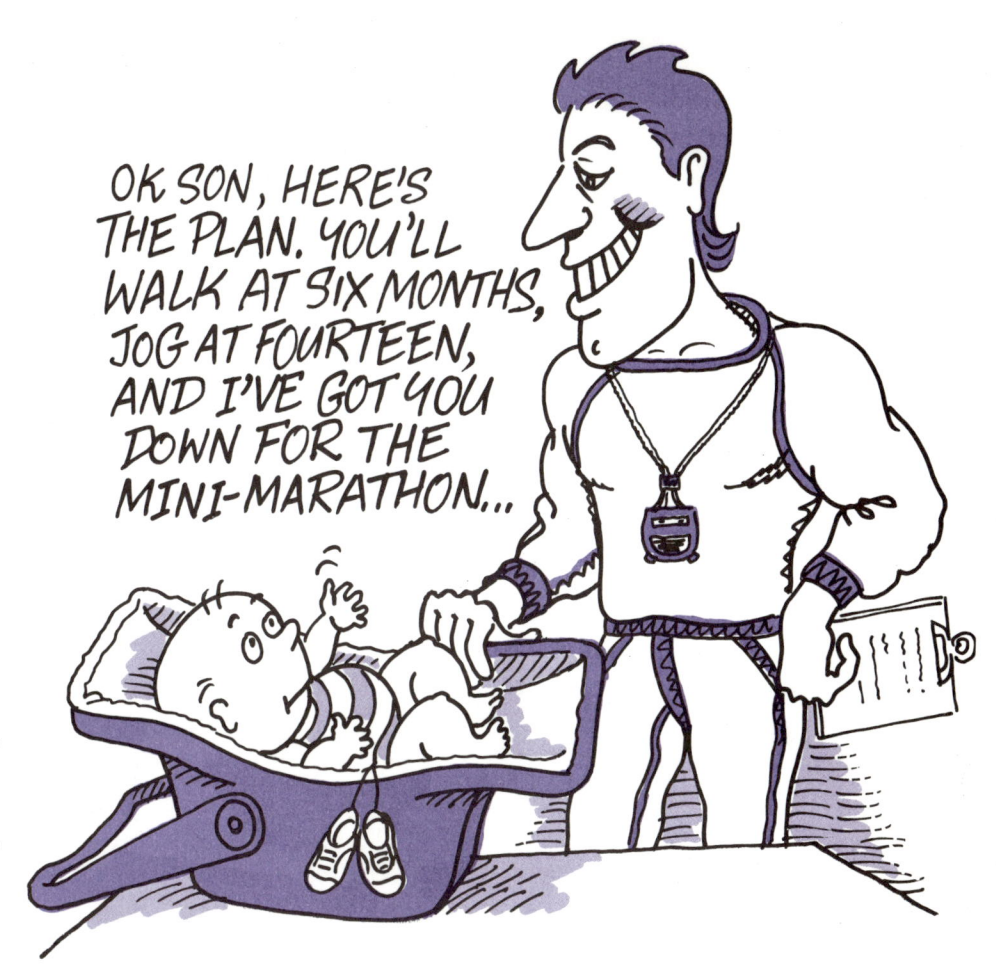

OK SON, HERE'S THE PLAN. YOU'LL WALK AT SIX MONTHS, JOG AT FOURTEEN, AND I'VE GOT YOU DOWN FOR THE MINI-MARATHON...

FATHERS GET ATTACHED TOO

As a young neonatologist, I once flew three hundred miles, as part of the Newborn Transport Team, from Denver to a small town in Kansas. We were to pick up a baby girl who had become sick within the first few days after birth. At the hospital I met and reassured the parents that we would stabilise her and then fly her back to Denver Children's Hospital in our aircraft. The little girl required an hour or so of stabilisation before we took off. As we wheeled the little girl in through the doors of the Denver hospital the father was there to greet us. He had beaten our flight to Denver in his car (and had received only one speeding ticket!) He watched over her cot until she was out of danger.

THE CIRCUMCISION DECISION

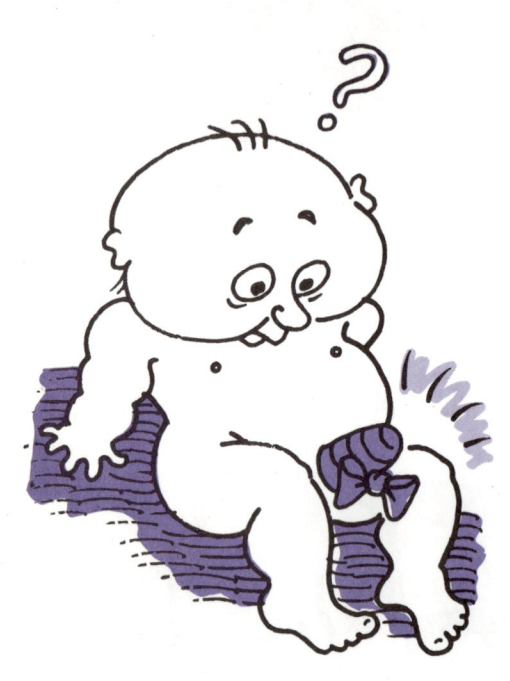

Most are aware that circumcision is an ancient Jewish ritual dating back to the time of Abraham, but few realise that the Jews were not the first to practise it. Carvings on the walls in the Temple of Karnak depict Egyptian priests over 6000 years ago performing circumcision, making it probably the oldest surgical operation known. Many diverse cultures continue the practice today.

In modern times circumcision became extremely popular between the wars – especially in the USA and Australia and rather less in the UK. The influential American paediatrician, Benjamin Spock, though not wholly recommending it, thought that 'it made a boy feel regular' as virtually all boys in that era were circumcised.

But times are changing.

Nowadays in the city obstetric hospitals over seventy per cent of male babies are going home still complete with foreskin – often to the dismay of their grandparents.

When the foreskin draws back
A common reason for excision of the foreskin in a baby is 'phimosis', that is narrowing of the foreskin. Many people – sadly including many medical and nursing professionals – are not aware that in the majority of baby boys the foreskin is not retractable. Only in four per cent of newborns can the foreskin be fully retracted. As time passes the foreskin gradually separates from the underlying tissue, but still by three years of age there are ten per cent of boys whose foreskin cannot be retracted. In these boys, as there is no space between the foreskin and the glans, no secretions collect and consequently there is no need for this area to be washed.

After the foreskin becomes retractable, such secretions do tend to accumulate and regular hygiene is necessary. Many misguided people forcibly retract the foreskin of the infant before it is ready and this in

IT'S NOT TRUE

With an ancient practice like circumcision it is not surprising that numerous myths have sprung up about its use. Circumcision apparently 'weakens the penis' and therefore limits intercourse (so said a twelfth century rabbi); increases (others say decreases) sexual pleasure; decreases sexual desire; prolongs ability to have intercourse; decreases the incidence of sexually transmitted disease; makes men better warriors and better husbands; reduces masturbation and cures bedwetting. These claims, as you can imagine, are difficult to research but all are unreasonable and defy commonsense.

Then medical opinion got in on the act and stated that circumcision decreased the incidence of cancer of the penis, and the wives of circumcised men had a decreased incidence of cancer of the cervix. Subsequent research showed both beliefs to be unfounded.

THE CIRCUMCISION DECISION

itself causes scarring and the subsequent possibility of narrowing (phimosis). This then makes retraction and normal hygiene extremely difficult. In fact to correct this situation, circumcision may be subsequently required. Most people who recommend circumcision have gruesome tales of close friends or relations who had 'years of infection, pain and worry' from a foreskin that was too narrow until they were liberated by circumcision. One wonders how many of these poor men were suffering from a consequence of obsessive early retraction and penile toilet when things would have been better left alone.

The function of the foreskin
Speaking purely logically, it seems likely that the foreskin has some function. Most of our other useless organs have been discarded by the process of evolution or remain only in a shrunken, vestigial form. Not so with the foreskin which remains as large as life. Examination of the foreskin cells with a microscope shows that it contains many sensory nerve endings relating to sexual excitation. It would therefore seem reasonable, if it were being removed for social reasons, to obtain the permission of the owner. At the age of twenty he should be able to make an informed decision. Moreover it is totally wrong to suggest that circumcision hurts more at that age. In fact it is not a particularly painful operation – as long as one has a general anaesthetic and there is no post-operative arousal!

It is certainly an advantage for a newborn to keep his foreskin to afford protection for the sensitive glans from the effects of nappy rash and the avoidance of meatal ulceration, a small painful ulcer which develops at the opening of the urethra only in the circumcised. Another common indication mooted for circumcision of the newborn is because the foreskin causes urinary obstruction. This is almost never the case and if it occurs at all it must be incredibly rare. Certainly ballooning of the foreskin on passing urine is a normal finding and is certainly not an indication for its removal.

The parents' decision
By far and away the most common indication for circumcision in the newborn period is parental preference. Parents often believe that it is the 'thing to do' and to leave their son uncircumcised would be to his later disadvantage. Fathers often wish their sons to be 'done' so that their penises and their sons' look the same. They are worried

If the baby's father and brothers are circumcised, most parents will want to have a matching set

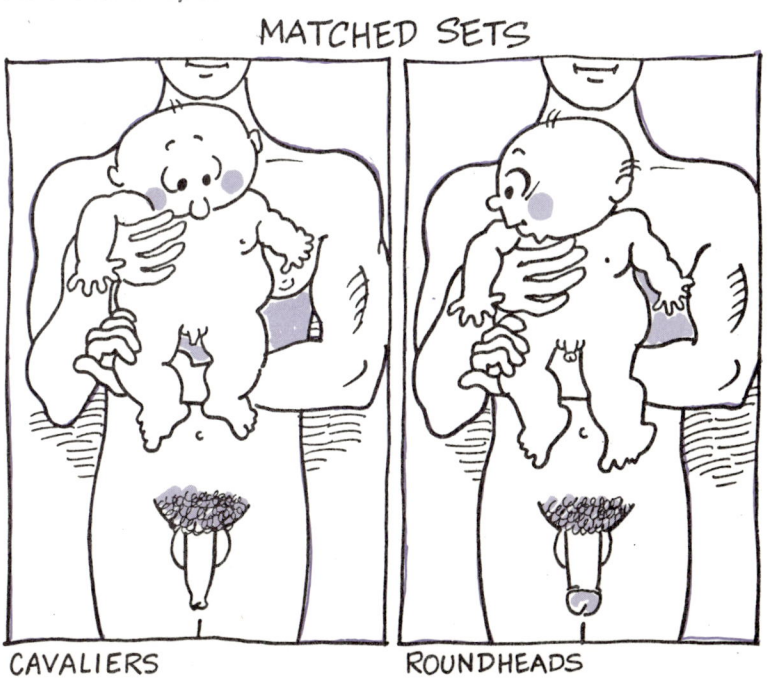

MATCHED SETS

CAVALIERS | ROUNDHEADS

THE CIRCUMCISION DECISION

It is safer to have an anaesthetic and a circumcision at about six months than an unanaesthetised neonatal circumcision

Recently a study has shown the possibility of an increased incidence of urinary tract infection in uncircumcised infants. This possibility is not yet proven and requires further confirmation. Certainly it has not changed the stance of the American Pediatric Association which is still firmly against the practice.

that any differences will cause the boy upset and confusion. Children, however, accept differences with far greater equanimity than do adults and the major difference between father and son, that of penile size, remains until he is well into puberty anyway. If the boy has brothers who are circumcised most parents seem to want a matching set, though again there is no evidence that differences cause any psychological harm.

The safest time for circumcision

A very important question and one which is only infrequently asked by parents is, what is the safest time for a baby to be circumcised? The answer to this is – the later the better. One thing is quite certain, the neonatal period (the first four weeks of life) is precisely the time when it is least safe. The newborn baby has immature immunity which makes him less than fully capable of fighting an infection should bacteria enter from his wound site. In addition, his clotting mechanisms are immature.

Most babies get jaundiced in the first few days of life and one of the reasons for this is immaturity of the liver. One of the functions of the liver is to process the jaundice and eliminate it from the body. Significantly, clotting factors are also produced by the liver. It certainly seems illogical to trust the clotting mechanism of a baby who has demonstrably immature liver function. The only advantage of circumcision in the newborn period is that, as the baby is so small, he can't fight back. It is felt, therefore, quite unjustifiably, that no anaesthetic is necessary. Nevertheless, it is safer to have an anaesthetic and a circumcision at about six months than it is to have an unanaesthetised neonatal circumcision.

Consequences

It is general knowledge in the paediatric community that occasionally babies die as a direct result of circumcision, with at least sixteen babies dying each year in the UK.

Other complications also occur. In a random study of a thousand families undertaken in England it was found that twenty-two per cent of the boys circumcised had developed some complication from the procedure and these included haemorrhages severe enough to require transfusion.

It must be said, however, that despite the risks associated with the age group of the patient, the operation would be a good deal safer if it was taken more seriously. Too frequently it is delegated to the junior member of an obstetric team. The operative area has a very good blood supply and luckily heals very quickly and it is difficult for an infection to gain a foothold. Also the skin is very mobile and if too much is removed usually this makes very little functional difference, so most irregularities in technique are of no consequence. Nevertheless, it is obvious that this part of the body is of tremendous psychological importance so, if mistakes are made, the scars remain not just on the body but in the mind.

THE SEAL OF APPROVAL

Every newborn infant should have a thorough physical examination early in his life. Such examinations are designed to detect any difficulties in adapting to life outside the womb and any congenital abnormalities or illnesses. During his stay in hospital the baby will usually have at least two or three physical examinations.

IN THE DELIVERY ROOM

As soon as a baby is born he will be examined:
- To assess any difficulty he may be encountering converting from a dependent life inside the womb, relying on the placenta for food and oxygen, to an independent life outside, utilising his lungs to obtain oxygen.
- To find any important congenital abnormalities that need immediate management and treatment.
- If all is well, and it usually is, to assure his terrified parents that they can stop worrying!

It is at this time that the Apgar score is done. Five physical signs of the baby are scored either zero, one or two to assess how well he's adapting to life outside the womb and whether he has been affected by delivery. The baby is assessed at one minute and five minutes after birth. A score of seven or more is normal but babies with lower scores usually do well.

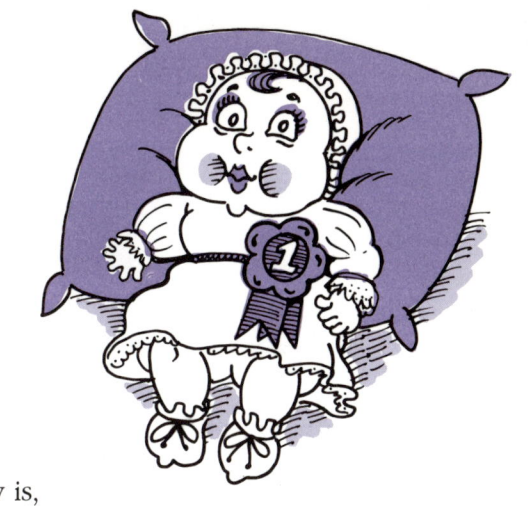

APGAR SCORE
performed at one and five minutes after delivery

	SCORE	0	1	2
S I G N S	Heart rate	Absent	Less than 100	More than 100
	Respiratory effort	Absent	Slow and irregular	Good and regular
	Muscle tone	Limp	Some flexion of limbs	Active motion
	Colour	Blue	Pink body, blue extremities	Completely pink
	Reflex response	Nil	Grimace	Cough or sneeze to nasal catheter

THE SEAL OF APPROVAL

When the baby has settled down and is warm, dry and comfortable, a paediatrician will examine him thoroughly.

Most birthmarks will disappear without treatment before your baby is five years old

FULL PHYSICAL EXAMINATION

A paediatrician can obtain lots of information about the baby merely by observing him. The baby usually lies in a relaxed posture with arms by his sides, elbows bent, hips and knees flexed. His body is straight with his head on one side. His colour is generally pink in Caucasian and Asian babies and rather darker in Negroid babies, although his hands and feet may be blue and cool for the first few days. After two or three days his colour may become slightly yellowish as the normal jaundice occurs. He breathes quietly at a rate of about forty breaths per minute but may also have the pattern of alternate panting and shallow breathing which is normal for the first three months of life. His face is examined to see whether it conforms to a normal appearance (if it seems a little unusual the paediatrician will usually have a look at dad before saying so!). Following this general look a more specific examination can be conducted.

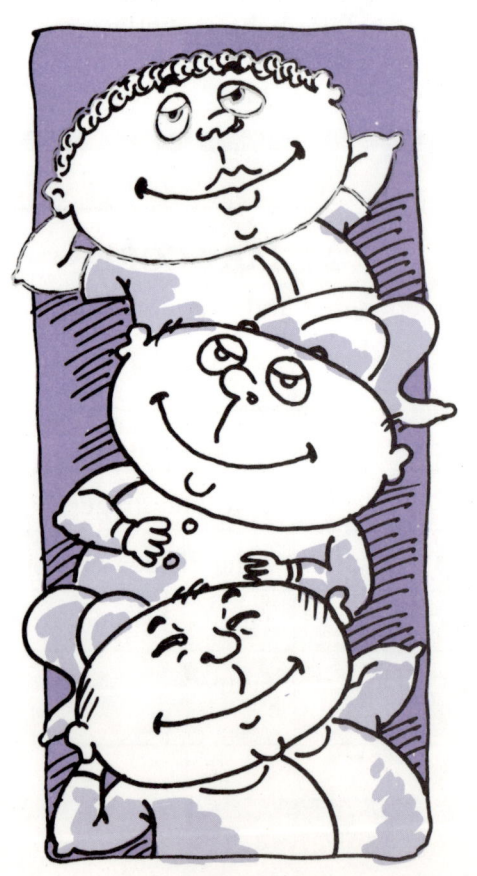

SKIN

Maturity
The thickness of the skin relates to the baby's maturity. A baby born early has fine, pink, delicate skin whereas the skin of a post-mature baby (a baby born two weeks or more after term) has a pale, scaly parchment-like appearance. White, greasy material, called vernix, may be present on the skin, especially in the creases, of all babies but particularly those born a week or two early.

Birthmarks
Most babies have got so-called 'stork-bites' which are flat red

THE SEAL OF APPROVAL

birthmarks over the eyelids, bridge of the nose and back of the neck. The ones on the face disappear over the first year.

Mongolian spots are irregular areas of deep blue pigmentation usually found above or around the buttocks. They occur in all races but especially in Asians and they mostly fade over the first few years.

More unusual are strawberry marks, which disappear without treatment before the age of five, and port-wine stains, which don't unless they are treated, usually with laser therapy.

Milia
These little white spots (like millet seeds – hence the name) are due to distended sweat glands and are mostly seen over the cheeks, chin, and nose. They are probably caused by the effect of hormones from the placenta on the developing sweat glands. Don't worry about

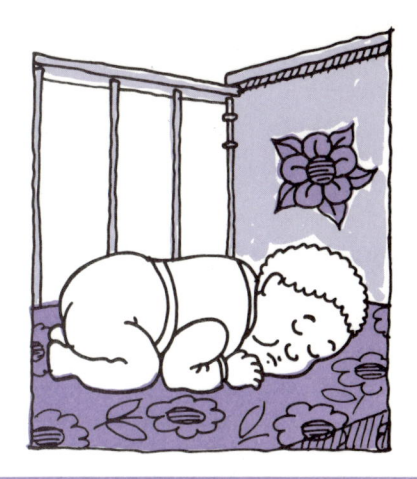

THE NEWBORN BABY

Newborns often worry their parents by their sometimes strange appearance. Most of these odd characteristics are quite normal and will disappear sooner or later.

• Swollen eyes	• Turned in feet
• A throbbing fontanelle	• Bowed legs
• Enlarged genitals	• Small, rather receding chin
• A rash of white spots over the face	• Blue hands and feet
• Changes in skin colour	• Swollen nipples
• A coating of greasy white vernix	• Ingrowing toenails
• Fine hair over various parts of the body, called lanugo	• Rubbery lumps under the skin, over the cheekbones and jaw
• Misshapen head, generally due to compression in the birth canal	• Swelling or bruising on the head as a result of labour
• Instrument marks if there was a forceps delivery	• Red marks over the eyelids, nose and back of neck

THE SEAL OF APPROVAL

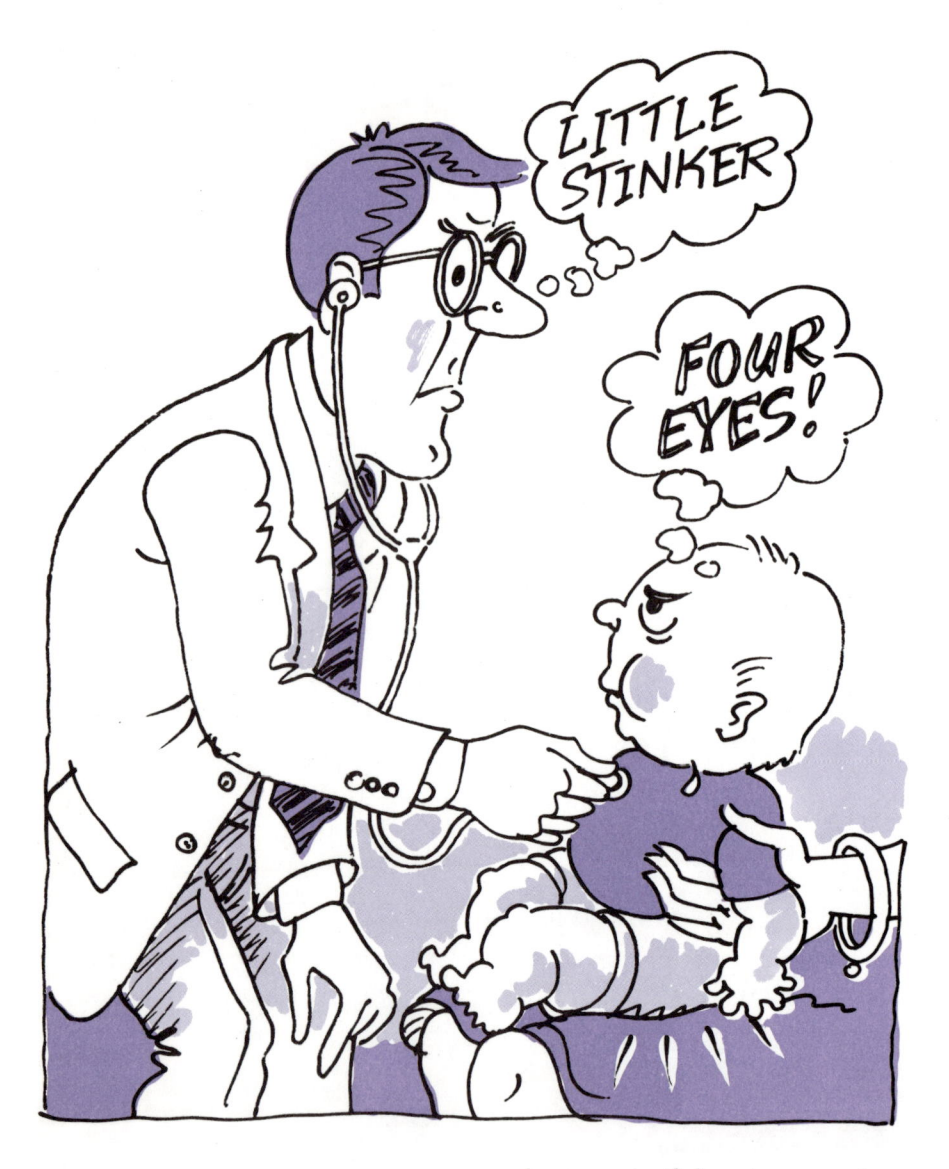

bad name quite unfairly. A forceps delivery is actually preferred by many paediatricians for premature babies. The forceps act as a protective cage around the soft skull. Used properly they do good, not harm. They are primarily used to guide the head of the baby through the lower part of the mother's pelvis if progress is slow or the head is in the wrong position or the mother is too tired to push.

THE HEAD

The paediatrician will measure the head circumference and feel the fontanelle and the edges of the skull bones.

The fontanelle is a diamond-shaped, soft spot at the top of the head which is easily indented with the finger. Despite its apparent vulnerability, it is a very thick, tough membrane and there is no danger at all of injuring your baby with normal handling. You may notice that it sometimes pulsates with the heartbeat or bulges when the baby cries or strains. This is normal. It often gets a little larger in the first few months, before closing between the age of nine and eighteen months.

Head shape

Babies are a bit like toothpaste in their ability to fit through tight places. Following delivery, particularly when the birth canal is narrow, the baby's head may be elongated and misshapen. This is very common and my only advice is to stop worrying and delay taking the first baby photographs.

Babies are designed very well for the journey down the

them, even if they increase in number, as they disappear after the first few weeks.

Forceps act as a protective cage around the soft skull. Used properly they do good, not harm

Other marks

Some babies have bruises and other marks from the delivery, especially on their heads and faces. Have no fear, babies are designed beautifully for what they have to go through and heal very rapidly. Within a couple of days most of the marks will have gone.

Don't get upset about forceps marks. This instrument has got a

THE SEAL OF APPROVAL

birth canal. In particular, the skull bones (of which there are four over the vault of the head) are not joined and can override each other to allow the head to pass down a narrow birth canal. This overriding, or molding, may be detected as thickening over the midline or above the ears following delivery. It disappears in the first few days and no harm can come to the brain underneath.

The head may also develop *caput*, which is a boggy irregular swelling of the soft tissues of the skull again due to compression by the birth canal during labour.

The bone may also become swollen. Bone has a membrane stuck firmly down to its surface and, during delivery, if a flat skull bone is flexed a little, this membrane may split off and there may be bleeding underneath. This gives a soft boggy swelling, called a *cephalhaematoma*, which takes a few weeks to disappear. In twenty per cent of cases, however, the swelling turns to bone and the skull shape remodels over a longer period of time, but it does disappear eventually.

THE EYES

These are usually blue/grey or brown and clear. Their final colour may not be obvious until the baby is about a year old. Small spots of blood within the white of the eye are very common and are due to the bursting of capillaries from compression during labour. They are completely harmless and disappear in a week or so. An intermittent squint is normal, especially when the baby feeds and, unless it is constant, there is no cause for concern. Parents should appreciate that their baby sees clearly from birth.

THE MOUTH

Small white cysts are frequently seen along the gum margins and on the hard palate, especially in the midline. They can be mistaken for thrush, are of no consequence and will soon disappear without treatment.

THE CHEST

Breast enlargement is seen in many infants and is of no significance. Sometimes there is a secretion of milky substance due to the stimulating effect of the hormones from the placenta. It is hardly necessary to examine the lungs with a stethoscope as a normal respiratory rate is by far the most sensitive index.

Babies see clearly from birth and can focus on your face from about twenty centimetres (or eight inches) away

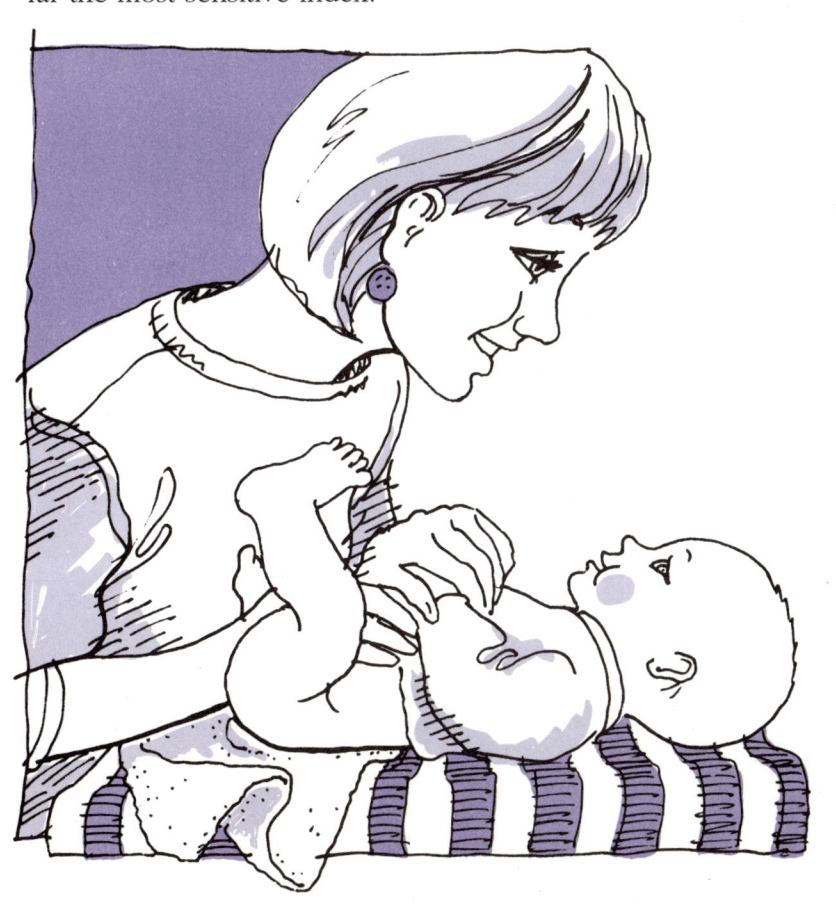

THE SEAL OF APPROVAL

SIGHT, HEARING, REFLEXES – THE NERVOUS SYSTEM

Throughout the examination, the posture, muscle tone, responses, moods, movements, and cry of the baby are observed and noted. He can be seen to turn to and gaze at light and will often stare fixedly at a face.

Hearing is somewhat more difficult to test in the first few days as the baby is very tolerant of loud noises. Remember he has just emerged from the noisy environment of the womb, with mother's aorta, the main artery of her body, banging away centimetres from his ear, her bowels gurgling and bladder filling and emptying. However, he can usually be made to respond to a clap or a loud noise if you catch him in the right mood.

THE REFLEXES

His reflexes will be tested. A baby is born with a number of automatic reactions to changes in his position or environment called 'primitive reflexes'. These are seen as a hangover from an early stage of man's evolution. These reflexes disappear over

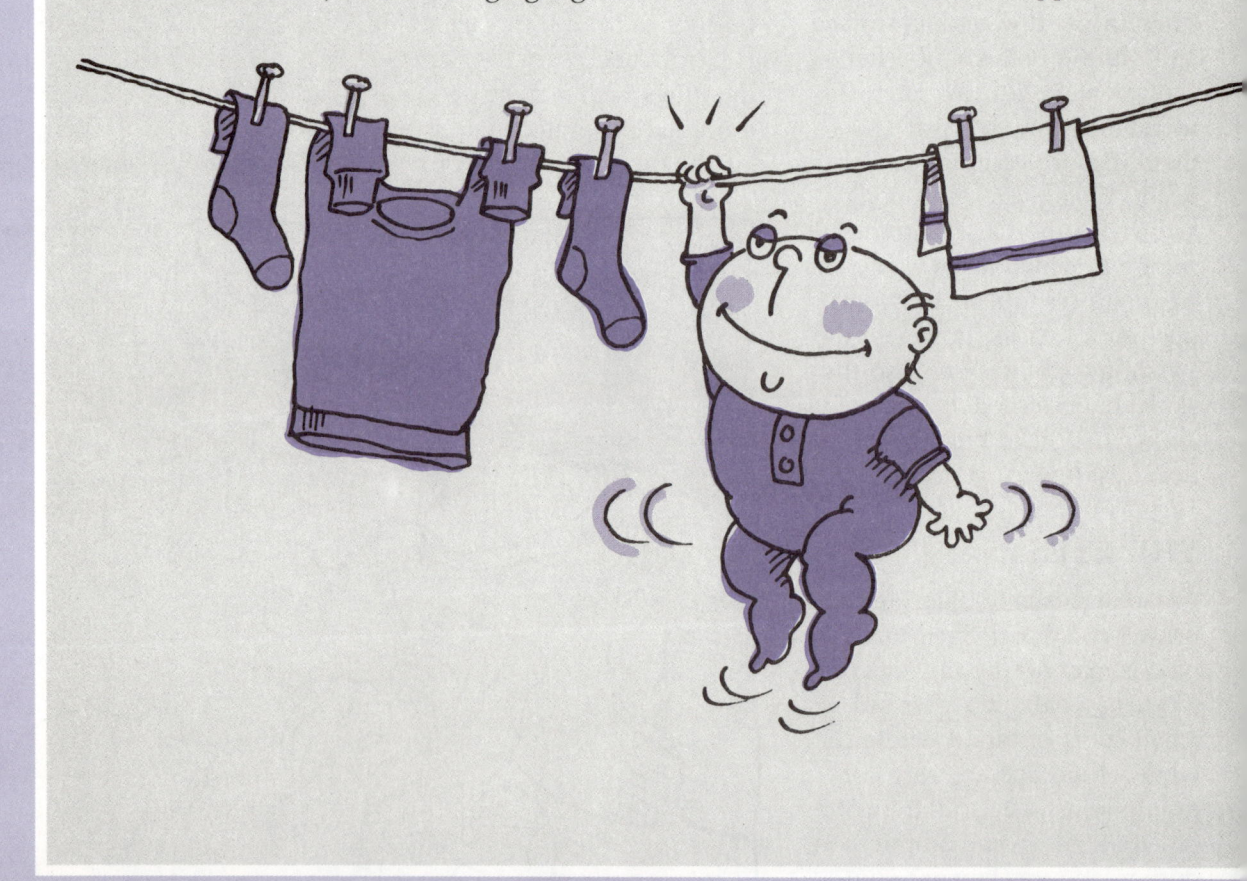

THE SEAL OF APPROVAL

the first weeks and months and by their disappearance, they indicate normal development of the baby's nervous system.

Especially obvious is his startle (Moro) reflex. If the baby's chin is positioned on his chest and his head is allowed to fall back, he will respond by flinging his arms out as if to grab at something. He will then move them in an arc towards the midline of his chest. At the same time he opens his eyes wide, looks unhappy, and may start to cry. A test of the Moro reflex is a good check of the baby's muscle tone. The reflex disappears gradually over the first two to three months.

Another reflex is his 'grasp' reflex. If you tickle his palm he will grip your finger. In fact he will automatically close his hand if something is placed in his palm. This reflex is so strong that a baby can actually support his body weight grasping two of your fingers. His toes will also flex in response to a similar stimulus to the sole of the foot.

If you brush your baby's cheek on one side he will turn his head in that direction. This is called the rooting reflex, and will ensure that he will root for the nipple when his cheek brushes against his mother's breast.

Proud parents often like to demonstrate their baby's 'walking' reflex. A baby, held in the standing position with feet on a flat surface, will make somewhat clumsy walking movements forward. This reflex disappears at about the age of four weeks.

The 'stepping' reflex is another interesting one. By bringing the baby's shin in contact with the edge of a flat surface, the leg will be raised to step over it as though he were climbing a staircase.

The 'Galant' reflex can be elicited by holding the baby over one hand, back towards you. By stimulating the lumbar region, for instance with a gentle scratch, the baby will curve his bottom towards the side of the stimulus.

THE HEART

The normal heartrate is usually between one hundred and one hundred and forty beats per minute. The heart is also checked with a stethoscope for the sound of a murmur. Most murmurs picked up in the first few days are quite harmless, due either to delay in the circulation changing from that of a fetus to that of a newborn, or the presence of tiny holes between the two main pumping chambers in the heart. Both of these problems right themselves within a short time and are harmless.

THE ABDOMEN

The doctor examines the abdomen to ensure the liver, spleen and kidneys are normal and feels for any abnormal lumps or masses. The umbilicus contains three vessels (one vein and two arteries). Occasionally an umbilical hernia (see page 37) may be present. This is of no significance as it rarely requires surgery and disappears by itself in time (usually by the age of five).

At the junction of the abdomen and the thighs, the main arteries to the legs are felt with the fingertips to exclude narrowing of the artery higher up.

THE GENITALS

These will be inspected carefully for any abnormalities.
In boys both testes are in the scrotum. Cold hands, however, may make them disappear temporarily as there is a reflex which pulls them up out of sight. Occasionally the testes are delayed on their journey down from the abdomen. They are

THE SEAL OF APPROVAL

Don't leave hospital worrying about a lot of unanswered questions

then termed undescended. Ninety per cent of these will descend on their own in the first year, the rest may require surgery to bring one or both into the scrotum.

In girls, the vulva looks rather swollen and red in comparison to later life. Mucus tags and occasionally bleeding may be seen at the opening of the vagina. Both occur because of stimulation from hormones from the placenta and neither is of any significance.

THE HIPS

The hip joints are examined for clicks, which are quite common in the newborn (and harmless), or dislocation. See later in this section for more on hips.

THE LEGS AND FEET

It is normal for babies to have bow legs. The slight curvature of the tibia is caused by their posture inside the womb. Most babies hold their feet turned inwards while in the womb and this may continue to be obvious for a few weeks after delivery. Occasionally this is called 'postural talipes' by some, but this is NOT club foot. If the foot can be held at right angles to the leg with the sole flat, then it is a normal ankle joint.

THE BACK

The doctor will check the spine to see that it is straight and has no faults. Very commonly there is a dimple at the base of the spine and this is quite normal and will grow out with time. The anus is also checked to see that it is open.

DISCHARGE EXAMINATION

Just before your baby goes home a final examination is performed. This is to check:
- The heart – to be sure no murmurs have emerged since the first examination. Because the baby's circulation is making great changes in these first few days some murmurs take a few days to develop.
- The head circumference is remeasured now that most of the molding has disappeared.
- The umbilical cord is checked for infection, and to make sure that the normal process of drying and separation is occurring.
- The baby's eyes are checked for 'stickiness' and, if necessary, tear duct massage taught to the mother.
- The skin is also examined for any rashes or pustules.
- The hips are rechecked just to be on the safe side. Those hips whose ligaments were marginally lax on the first day should now be much firmer in their sockets and, if so, can be safely left alone but carefully followed up.
- The feeding is assessed to see if it is going well. The baby is usually weighed – though at this stage whether or not there is any gain doesn't mean much.
- Any questions you have can be answered. Now is the time to clear up any conflicting advice you may have been given, and to find out how to get help if things start to worry you after you go home. Don't waste the opportunity! On the next page are some of the questions most commonly asked.

QUESTIONS AND ANSWERS

Being a first-time mother is by definition a new experience, full of tasks to be learned and problems to be solved. In the light of this, there is no such thing as a stupid question. Use these questions as the basis for your own list, writing down any others as they occur to you.

Q. If he vomits some of his feed, should I top him up again?

A. That depends on him. If he appears willing to suck, top him up and if he does not seem to mind, wait for him to demand before putting him back on the breast.

Q. When should I take him to see the Health Centre Nurse?

A. First babies should probably go weekly to start with until weight gain is established, then as often as mother wishes. For subsequent babies, fortnightly visits are usually enough.

Q. How do I know when my baby has had enough at a feed?

A. He will stop sucking and may fall asleep but not necessarily. If he does, don't wake him by burping him, put him down in his cot.

Q. How do I handle the stump of his umbilical cord? Will it bleed? When and how will it heal up and fall off?

A. Remember that your baby cannot feel pain from his umbilical cord so handling it will cause him no discomfort. Give it a gentle tug when cleaning it to get down into the gutter. Cords often bleed a little in the days after birth but it is usually only backflow from the clotted veins within the cord and is of no significance. The umbilical cord heals up by becoming gummy and separating at the base, this process can take between 4 days and 6 weeks.

Q. Should I clean my baby's ears? Is there a safe way to do it?

A. It is not a good idea to immerse your baby's ears in water as the canal is difficult to dry and can get infected. Clean only the ear you can see. Do not poke anything in the ear canal.

Q. If my baby gets a rash, should I go on bathing him and with what?

A. Don't use soap on the affected area. Use a non-soap cleanser or pine tar solution in his bath. It's not necessary to bathe him every day. First babies get bathed every day, second babies alternate days and fourth babies twice a week!

Q. How many wet nappies should I expect my baby to have each day?

A. Babies who are being well fed may have between five and twelve wet nappies a day. If he has only two, let your doctor or midwife know.

Q. Should I clean the baby's genital area and how? Should I draw back the foreskin or should I leave it alone?

A. Do not draw back the foreskin until it has separated from the glans underneath when it will become easy to retract. This may take one year or more. Take your lead from your little boy, he will play with it in his bath and show you how far back it can comfortably be retracted. For little girls, gentle spreading of the outer lips and drawing a wet cottonwool ball from front to back within the vulva is often necessary. The vagina is self-cleaning.

THE SEAL OF APPROVAL

Babies quite commonly are born with a condition called 'clicky hips' and far less commonly, with a congenital dislocation of the hip.

Most newborns are 'double jointed' and their hips, which have ball-and-socket joints, have a fair amount of give between the ball and the socket

Many mothers have heard of 'clicky hips' but few have a clear idea what this means. Indeed, even doctors who study the subject closely are still in the dark about some aspects of this condition.

One of the many functions of the female hormones produced by the placenta is to soften mother's ligaments to make the birth of the baby easier. These hormones cross the placenta and have a similar effect on the newborn baby. Consequently, most newborns are 'double jointed' and their hip joints, which are ball-and-socket joints, have a fair amount of give between the ball and the socket. This is, of course, a normal phenomenon. However, in some babies this looseness may represent not just lax ligaments but the possibility of developing an abnormally shallow socket.

It is most important that babies who will develop shallow sockets are discovered as early on in life as possible so that treatment to form a normally deep socket can be started. This condition, even at its worst, is curable but only if we can spot these babies before the age of six months. We call the condition 'congenital dislocation of the hip' or CDH.

We know that, especially in girls, certain groups of babies are more likely to have this propensity. These are:
- those with a family history of congenital dislocation of the hip
- breech births
- babies who had only a small amount of amniotic fluid
- babies who have other evidence of a cramped environment in the uterus
- babies who are found to have clicky hips on examination following birth

The examination of baby's hips should always be done by someone skilled at detecting CDH. It involves holding the hip firmly at right angles to the axis

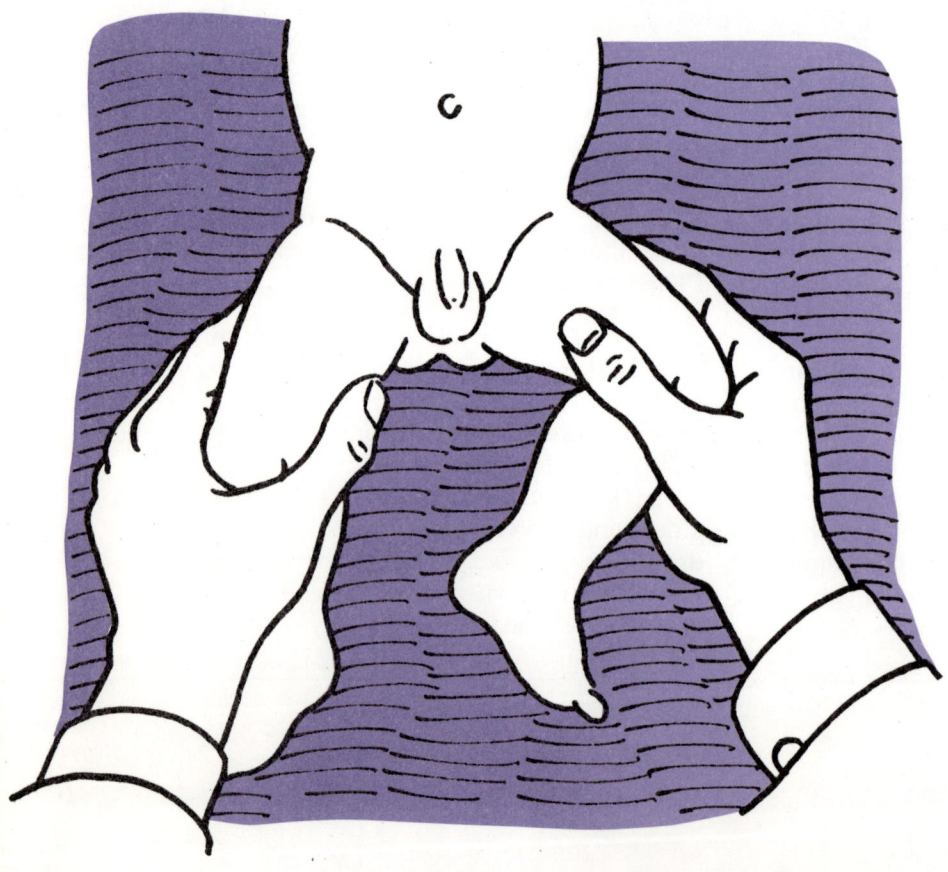

THE SEAL OF APPROVAL

of the body with the baby on his back facing the examiner, who then gently attempts to push the ball of the leg bone (femur) backwards out of the socket. Having done that, the leg is then rotated outwards so the baby is in a 'frog' posture. This tests the stability of the joint to dislocation.

If the head of the femur can be persuaded to leave the socket or there is excess give in the joint, most paediatricians prescribe a 'Pavlik harness'. This is a device of straps and Velcro which holds the hips up at right angles to the axis of the body – not in the frog posture like some old-fashioned devices. All this one does is stop the baby stretching his legs out. He is free to move the knees apart or together.

This harness is a bit of a nuisance but that is all. It is difficult to bath your baby completely as the harness must not be removed at all for the first weeks. But you'll all quickly get used to it after a week or so and usually it'll only be on for about twelve weeks. When it comes off, your baby's hips will be normal for the rest of his life – so it's worth it.

For all of these babies and any others in the 'high risk' groups, it is important to get a single hip X-ray at the age of five months. Ultrasound can be used at an earlier age, but the test is not yet used commonly. Before five months the hip joint is made only of cartilage, not bone, so unfortunately the X-rays cannot show the joint properly. X-ray alone will be able to exclude CDH and, though it is an unusual condition, it is critical that it be found no later than this age.

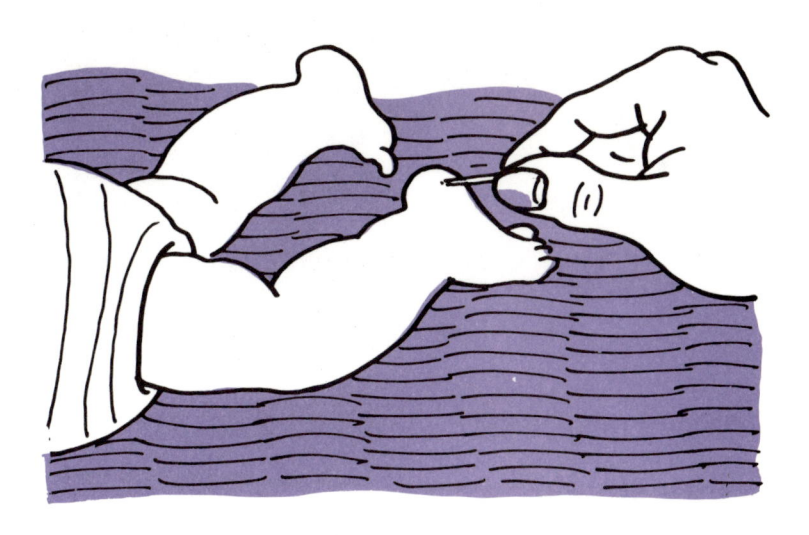

In the first few months, there is another useful physical sign of the possible presence of CDH. When the baby is lying on his back on his change table, normally the hips can be spread apart so that the knees can touch the surface of the table (or nearly). If it feels like there is a block to that movement, it is worth getting your paediatrician to examine your baby's hips, just to be on the safe side.

THE GUTHRIE TEST

The Guthrie test is a blood test performed on your baby in the first week after birth. A blood sample is taken by a heel prick and the blood absorbed onto a special piece of blotting paper. The sample is dried and sent to a central laboratory for testing. This screening test is designed to pick out those very few babies who have some rare diseases called 'inborn errors of metabolism'. That is, they are born missing some functions to do with the breakdown of food into the building blocks of the body and/or the building up of body tissues from those building blocks. These disorders are extremely rare (one in thirty thousand to a hundred thousand population).

The Guthrie test these days incorporates two other very important tests:
- Thyroid function – the test will pick up if your baby's thyroid is not producing enough hormone (this is an important cause of brain damage if it is not picked up immediately).
- Cystic fibrosis – this is a disease of the excreting glands of the body which has important effects in the baby's lungs and digestive system.

You are not informed of a negative result of these tests. However, it is not unusual for the laboratory to ask for a further sample in the case of a borderline result or laboratory problems. Overwhelmingly, under these circumstances the test will be negative and they will inform you of the result of this repeat test as soon as it is done. If the test happens to be positive you will hear about it soon after the test is done.

EARLY DAYS

It is important to remember, when we read so much about what can go wrong during pregnancy and childbirth, that most babies are born free of problems. Occasionally, there may be some early difficulties, most of which will be quite quickly resolved.

Small babies should still be immunised at the usual time – eight to twelve weeks from their birth date

SMALL BABIES

Babies who weigh less than 2.5 kg (5 lbs) at birth are defined as small. Smallness can be due to:
- Having small parents. In this case the baby would behave and have the same needs as any other term baby.
- Prematurity. Such a baby may have immaturity of some important functions, resulting in poor sucking and feeding, respiratory difficulty, a tendency to get cold easily, for the blood sugar level to drop and general lethargy.
- 'Small for Dates.' This baby is more mature than his weight implies but he is undernourished, usually because the placenta, and hence food transferral from mother, did not function well in the final weeks.

Babies in the last two groups are given extra attention by the staff until they are stable and functioning as a larger baby might. Obviously if the babies are very small, unstable or require special care for any reason, they are admitted into a neonatal intensive care unit. Their management is beyond the scope of this book, however, suffice it to say that the vast majority of babies admitted to such units do very well and, if premature, will generally be home by the time they are thirty-eight weeks gestation.

Observations
Small babies who are, however, big enough to stay with their mother in the postnatal ward are

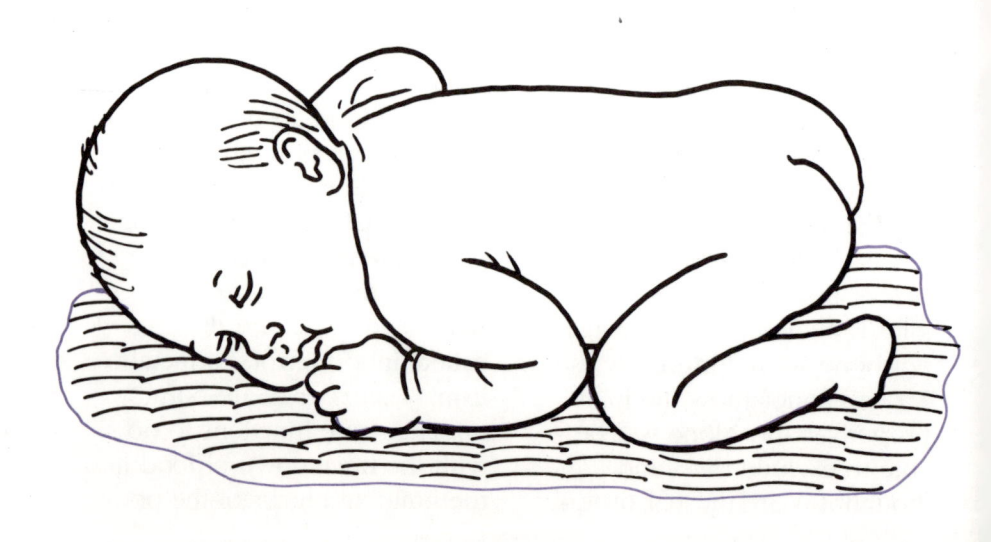

EARLY DAYS

regularly observed by nursing staff with observations of respiratory rate, heart rate and temperature every four hours. They also have regular heel-prick tests with Dextrostix or BM sticks, to measure the blood sugar level.

Management

If the baby is a week or so premature (that is thirty-five to thirty-six weeks gestation) mother can expect feeding to take a little longer to establish, as the suck reflex may not be at full strength for a few days. It can require a lot of patience and determination to stick to breastfeeding with some of the slower ones.

In contrast, the 'small for dates' baby may have a voracious appetite and work hard to put on the weight he feels is his birthright – at his poor mother's expense. Again, patience! When his weight catches up (usually within the first three months) he'll suddenly settle down to a more relaxed schedule. It is worth remembering that these babies have poor stores of energy for the first few days. This means:
- An eye must be kept on their blood sugar level until it is stable. This is easily monitored with regular checks of heel-prick blood.
- They may require complementary feeds of formula if they are too small to wait for the arrival of the breast milk in two or three days.
- Their temperature must be checked regularly as babies can chill easily if inadequately dressed in a cool environment.

Small babies should still be immunised at the usual time – eight to twelve weeks from their birthdate.

THE EMPTY-HANDED MOTHER

It is pretty depressing if your baby needs to be in the special care nursery instead of by your side. Quite apart from the anxiety, there is often a feeling that you have let him down because you cannot meet all of his needs by yourself and that in some way your bonding with your baby will suffer (properly managed, it will not).

Special care nurseries seem to evoke different responses in different parents. Some find the technology reassuring, they feel that all the equipment is really making their baby better. Others are just terrified that their baby needs to be looked after in an environment that seems more suitable for an astronaut than their precious baby.

The staff will encourage you to spend as much time as possible with your baby and if this feels comfortable, do it. If, on the other hand, sitting by him terrifies and panics you, do not feel compelled to do so. After a few days you will feel comfortable enough to stay with him for longer and longer periods. There are no hard and fast rules.

Many parents, especially mothers, go through a brief period much like grieving if their baby has a problem after birth. They grieve for the loss of the perfection they imagined during the pregnancy. They may feel disappointment and anger, as well as sadness and anxiety, as they struggle to adjust. These powerful emotions are either di-

Mothers grieve for the loss of the perfect baby they imagined during pregnancy

EARLY DAYS

rected inwardly, as guilt, or outwardly, as anger towards the partner, staff and even baby.

Like every other part of the body, our mind also has to heal when it has been injured, and these emotions are a part of the healing process. Accept them for what they are – a painful but important pathway to feeling better. They will pass and, for the vast majority of mothers, be replaced by joy as the healthy baby is placed in her arms.

FIRST DAY MUCUS

Many babies vomit a lot of mucus in the first twenty-four to forty-eight hours. The mucus is produced by the stomach lining as a reaction to delivery. It may be continually produced in excess for a day or two, so washing out the stomach with a tube does no good. The mucus, which may be blood-stained, as well as being vomited up, sometimes also makes the baby reluctant to feed.

This mucus is also the commonest cause of 'blue turns' during this period. It can be very thick, like treacle, and can cause temporary obstruction to the baby's breathing. This usually gives mothers quite a fright but it is important to remember that the baby's breathing drive and cough reflex are very powerful and he will be able to cough the obstruction out of the way without help. There is no need for any special treatment, but tipping the baby onto his side and patting his back seems to be the usual response.

STICKY EYES

About fifteen per cent of babies develop sticky eyes within a few days of birth. One or both eyes start to discharge mucus or pus from under the lids. It can be so profuse as to gum the lids together, especially after the baby has been asleep for a while.

Facts
- Rarely does the baby have conjunctivitis. Ninety-nine times out of a hundred he does not have a contagious infection which can be passed either to the other eye or to you.
- The baby's sight will not be affected.
- What the baby has is a blocked tear duct.

If you look at the inner corner of your eye, you will be able to see a fleshy bead-shaped structure. This is the tear sac, which collects the tears secreted by the eye, and passes them down a narrow tube (the tear duct) to the cavity of your nose. That's why your nose runs when you cry.

In babies there is a tendency for the bottom end of this duct to become blocked with a little plug of mucus. There is then a nice warm test tube of tears which incubates and grows whatever germs happen to be around at the time, and this produces the pus. The problem will disappear when the plug at the bottom of the tube is cleared by the body's normal processes, but until then it requires a little treatment. Pressing gently with

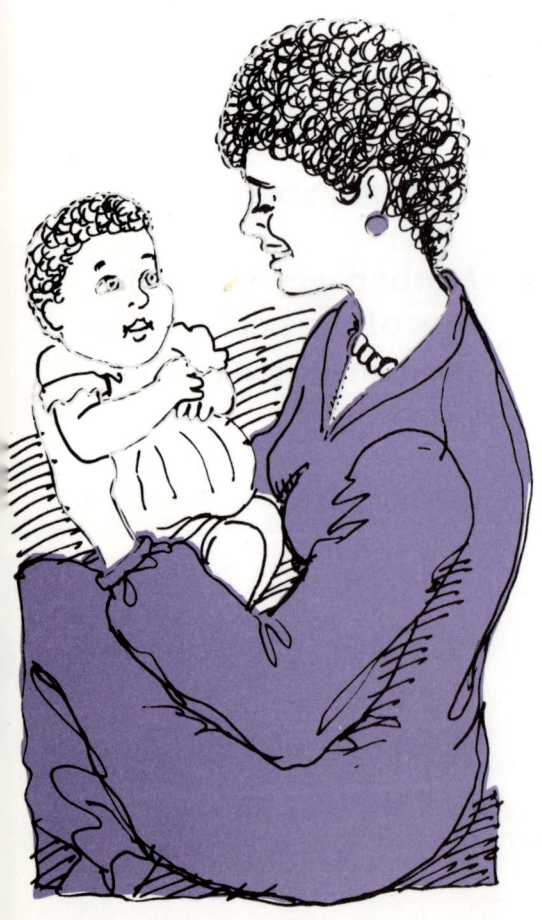

EARLY DAYS

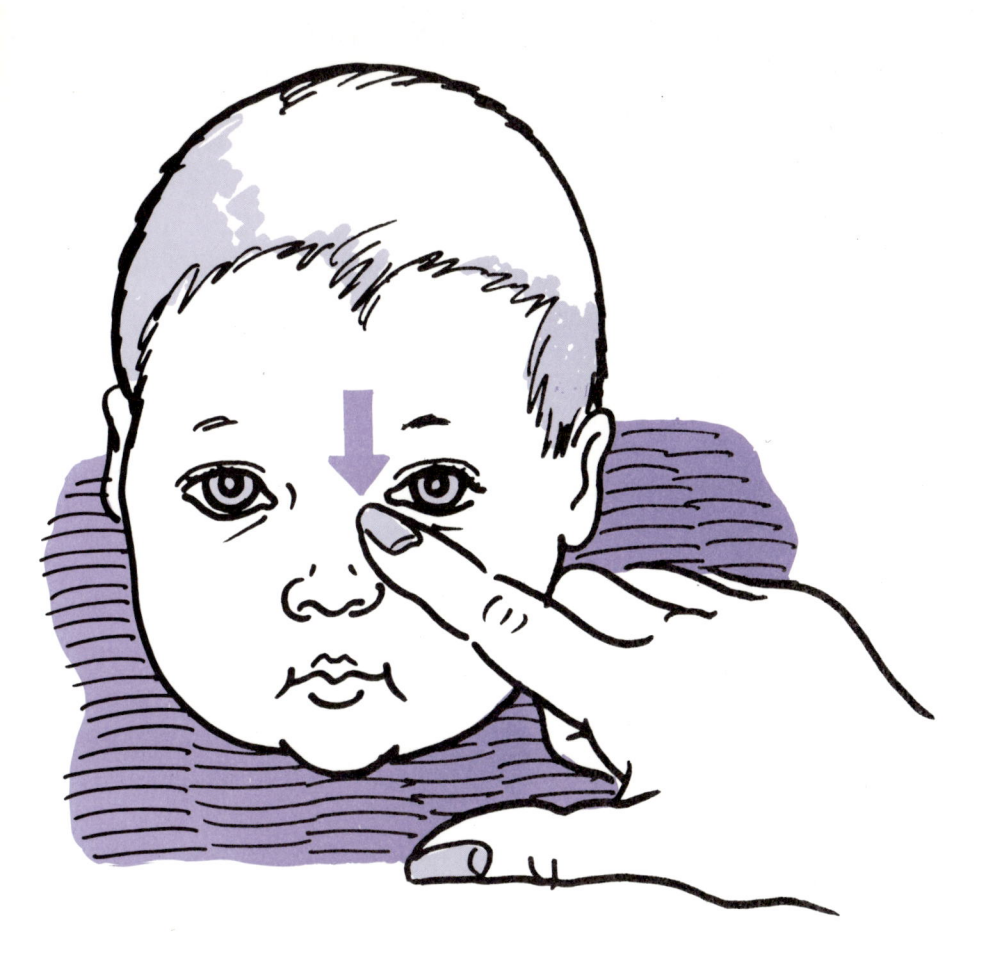

Massaging the tear duct as shown in this illustration is the ideal treatment for sticky eyes

the fingertip from the inner corner of the eye to half way down the side of the nose will squeeze out fluid and pus from both ends of the tear duct. Do this for ten strokes three times a day. Then clean the eye, ideally with saline but cooled, boiled water will do. If the eye becomes very gummy it is often helpful to instil some antibiotic eyedrops which can be prescribed for you by your doctor. This does not cure the condition but tends to cut down the number of germs within the tear duct and stops dried pus from making the mucus plug even more difficult for the body's normal mechanisms to remove.

The tear duct massage should be continued until the eye has been clear for a few days. It is only rarely that the problem lasts for more than a few days and if it does, the treatment is just the same. Only if the stickiness and weeping of the eye continue for six months or more does probing of the duct by an ophthalmologist have to be considered. Even then, delaying the probing still longer usually results in the tear duct clearing itself quite spontaneously.

INGROWING TOENAILS

Many babies are born with very short toenails, especially on the big toes. The nails are quite normal and grow out without any problem. Occasionally, as

Tear duct massage should be continued until the eye has been clear for a few days

31

EARLY DAYS

the nails grow, the skin against the nail's leading edge becomes red and inflamed. All that is required is a little local antiseptic for a week or so. Even if the skin starts developing crusty granulations it still requires no further treatment. Only the most severe cases need antibiotics or referral to a surgeon.

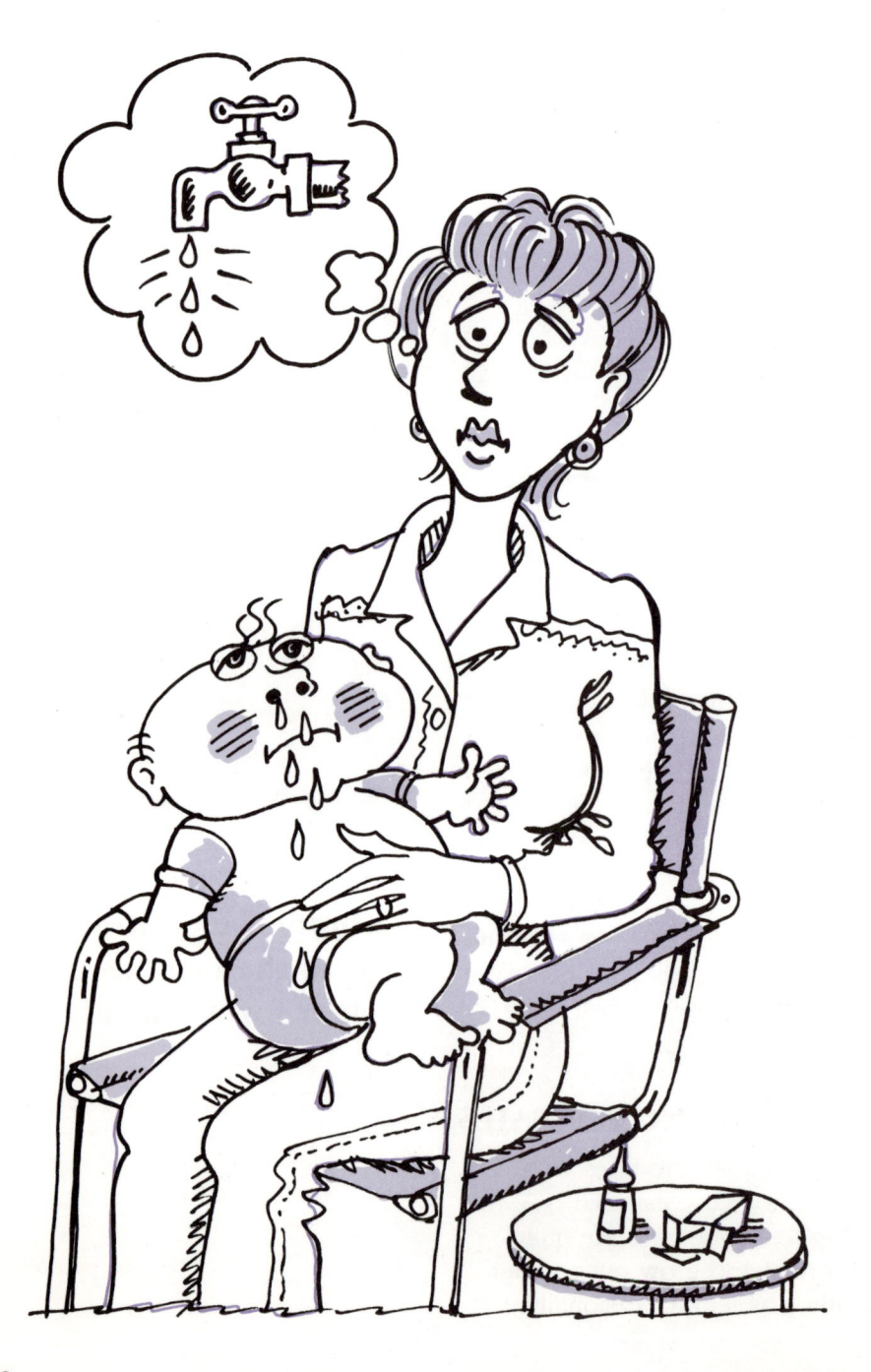

SNUFFLES

Eight out of ten babies get fairly heavy snuffles in the first few days. Don't worry, the baby does not have a cold. The delicate lining of the nose is producing lots of extra mucus to protect itself from an onslaught of milk and, if the baby regurgitates, gastric juice. When babies start to feed they are not particularly efficient about whether the milk goes down into the gullet or up into the nose so this problem is pretty common. If the snuffles are interfering with the baby's sleeping or feeding, local decongestant nasal drops can be helpful but, a word of warning, your baby will hate it. You will therefore be given a moving target and the nose is a pretty small target anyway.

My advice is to ignore the snuffles and they will go away. Occasionally, the amount of mucus produced by the nose can be so great that it pours out of the back of the nose and down into the pharynx where it collects in the throat and gives the baby a 'rattly chest'. Again, this is nothing to worry about. If your baby really catches a cold he is likely to have not only snuffles or a cough, but a raised temperature and will appear unwell. You will know that he is just not himself – this is not the case with a mere snuffle.

TOXIC ERYTHEMA

'There are fleas in this hospital – and they're biting my baby'

A day or so after delivery it is common for a baby to suddenly come out with a skin rash that makes him look rather like he

EARLY DAYS

has been attacked by fleas or mosquitoes. The rash has a yellowish head surrounded by a wide red area. Occasionally there may be many such spots, which all run together making the baby look like he's got the measles. This rash is called 'toxic erythema' and is completely harmless and not the least toxic! It seems to relate to the baby's skin first coming into contact with clothes, especially cotton. It does not mean the baby is allergic to anything nor that he has particularly sensitive skin. The rash will go away after a few days and does not cause discomfort.

HICCUPS

You probably noticed your baby was hiccupping in the womb and now he hiccups outside. It tends to occur during or after feeds and these enormous hiccups rack his little body like convulsions! Don't worry. It is a sign of gratitude for a good feed and no treatment is necessary.

DRY SKIN

Most babies born at term, and all babies born post-maturely, develop dry skin in the days after delivery. At its most obvious the skin can have deep cracks and fissures and the baby may slough off sheets of dead skin like a snake. More usually, though, the skin just gently scales and peels, especially over the hands and feet.

The top layer of skin that has been in contact with the amniotic fluid is merely being replaced and:
• it doesn't mean the baby will have a permanently dry skin;
• it has no relationship to eczema; and
• it needs no treatment. However, moisturising with sorbolene, for example, will make the baby's skin look a little more like the proverbial baby's bottom!

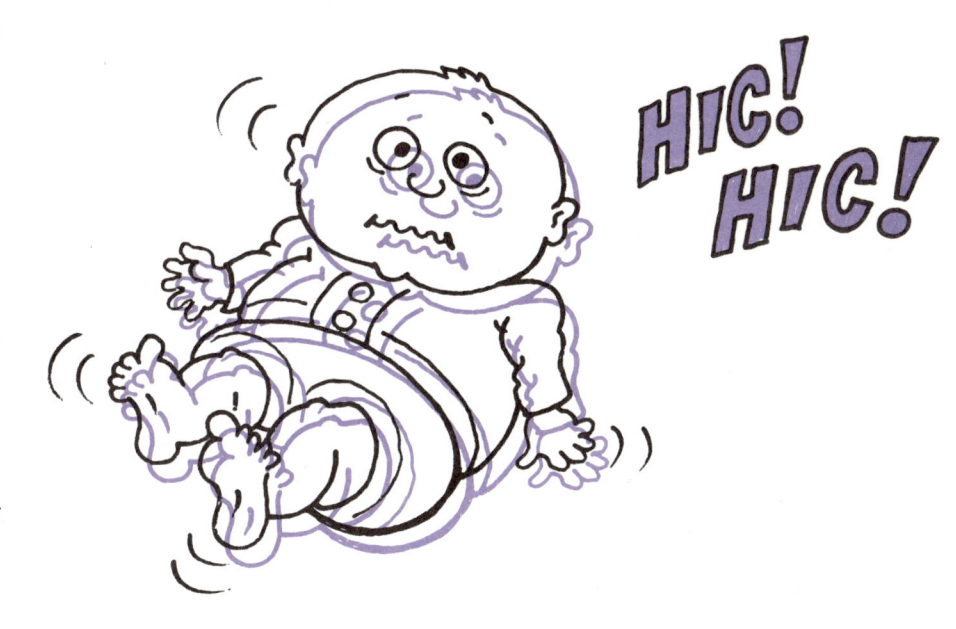

PINK-STAINED NAPPIES

Sometimes mothers get a fright when they change their baby's nappy – the urine appears to be bloodstained! In fact, it is not blood but a pinkish staining chemical, called 'urate', which babies pass in high concentration for the first few days after delivery. It is quite normal.

Little girls sometimes do have bloodstained nappies. A proportion of baby girls actually menstruate following the withdrawal of the hormones they had from the placenta. If they don't actually produce blood, most of them will produce a vaginal discharge in the first few days

Moisturising dry skin with sorbolene will make it more like the proverbial baby's bottom

EARLY DAYS

and this is quite normal. Many girls will also have a mucus tag hanging from the back of the vagina. This is also caused by stimulation from the hormones from the placenta and disappears after a few days.

GOOD URINARY STREAM

While we are on the subject of nappies, most little boys show their respect for their mother at an early stage by weeing over her. This 'shower' offers you a chance to make a worthwhile observation! It means the baby's urinary stream is perfectly normal. If the urine just dribbles out of the little boy it is a good idea to let your paediatrician or midwife know. Occasionally they can have flaps in their urinary passage from the bladder, which prevents a good stream and can cause problems if left untreated. This problem does not occur in little girls.

FOURTH-DAY BLUES

The fourth day is a bitch. Your milk has just come in and you have these two beach balls on your chest. Your baby is slightly jaundiced and you don't know what is going on with him. He has been feeding two-hourly for the last twenty-four hours and you can't remember ever feeling so tired before. The newness and delight of the birth is starting to fade and you feel just plain depressed. Everyone who comes to see you does nothing but look at the baby and tell you how wonderful you must be feeling. Your bottom is sore and you can't sit comfortably or,

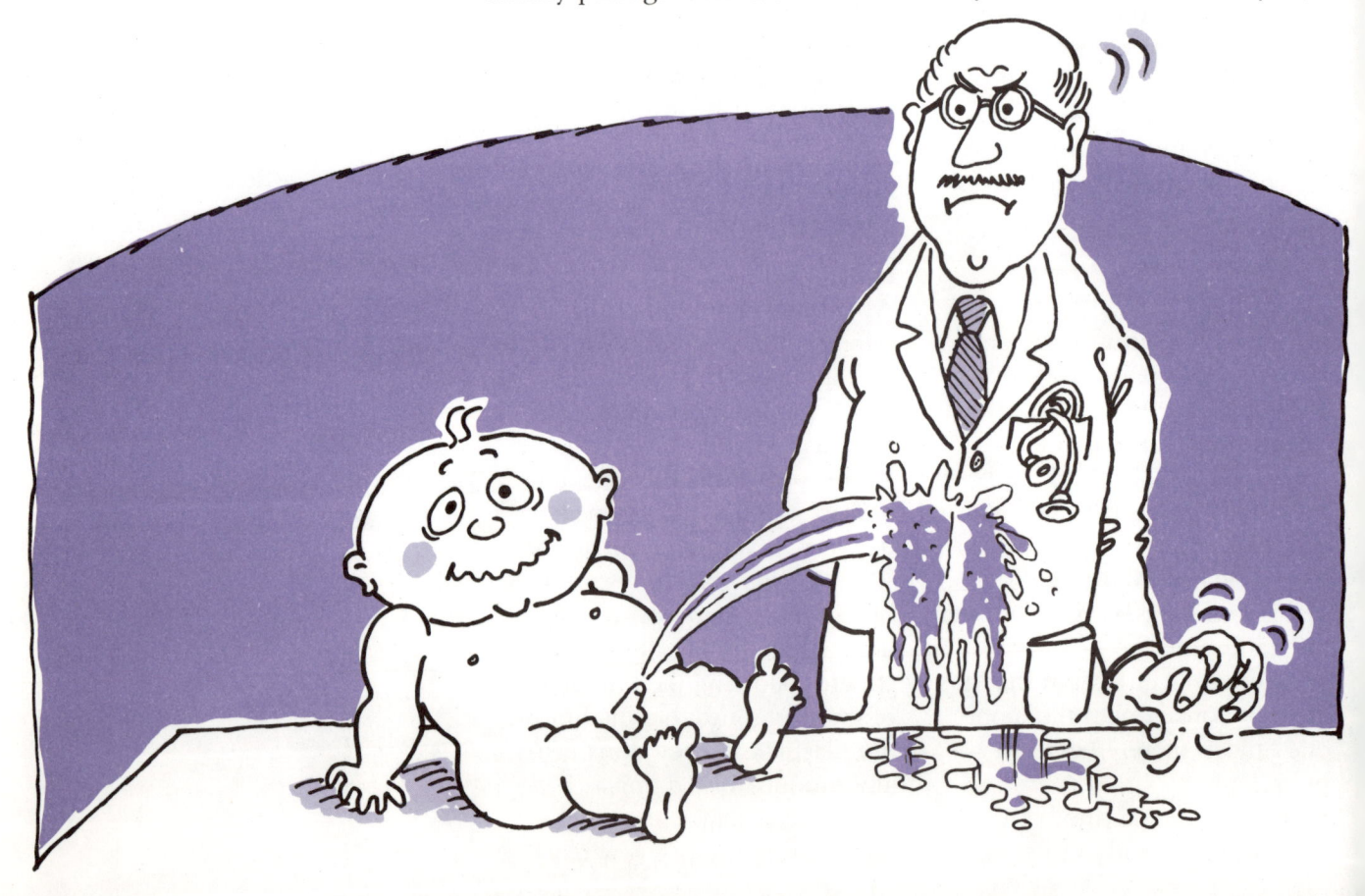

Many little boys wee all over Mum or the doctor. This indicates the baby has a normal urinary stream

EARLY DAYS

if you had a Caesarean, your incision hurts. On top of that, opening your bowels is difficult and very painful.

The only comforting thing to say about this picture of woe is that most mothers go through it. It seems to be related to the withdrawal of the high levels of placental hormones which were, believe it or not, putting you on a 'high' during your pregnancy. Day four seems to bring all these things to a head and my recommendation is to find a quiet corner (the shower is a popular choice) and have a good cry.

Sometimes this depression can last several days or even longer, but that is unusual. If it seems to be happening to you, do not keep it to yourself. It is important, will be taken seriously and it can be treated. It is also probably more common than women let on.

Many of the problems with the baby seem to explode out of all proportion today. He seems to have an insurmountable feeding problem. You suspect his jaundice is not the normal type but some new disease. When he cries, he seems to be blaming you for being born and you are sure all the doctors and nurses think you're a lot of trouble. The fact that your commonsense tells you that all this is untrue is not much help. Hang in there – these feelings will soon pass.

FEVERS

Many babies have a little fever on day two or three and this does not represent infection or any problem. It usually coincides with the baby being at his driest, that is, after he has lost the extra water in his body and before the milk has come in. At this age babies are very susceptible to overwrapping. So make sure, if the weather is warm, that he does not have too much covering him. As a rule, babies should be dressed in the same number of layers and thickness of clothing as you are. Babies do not need specially warm clothes unless conditions are very cool.

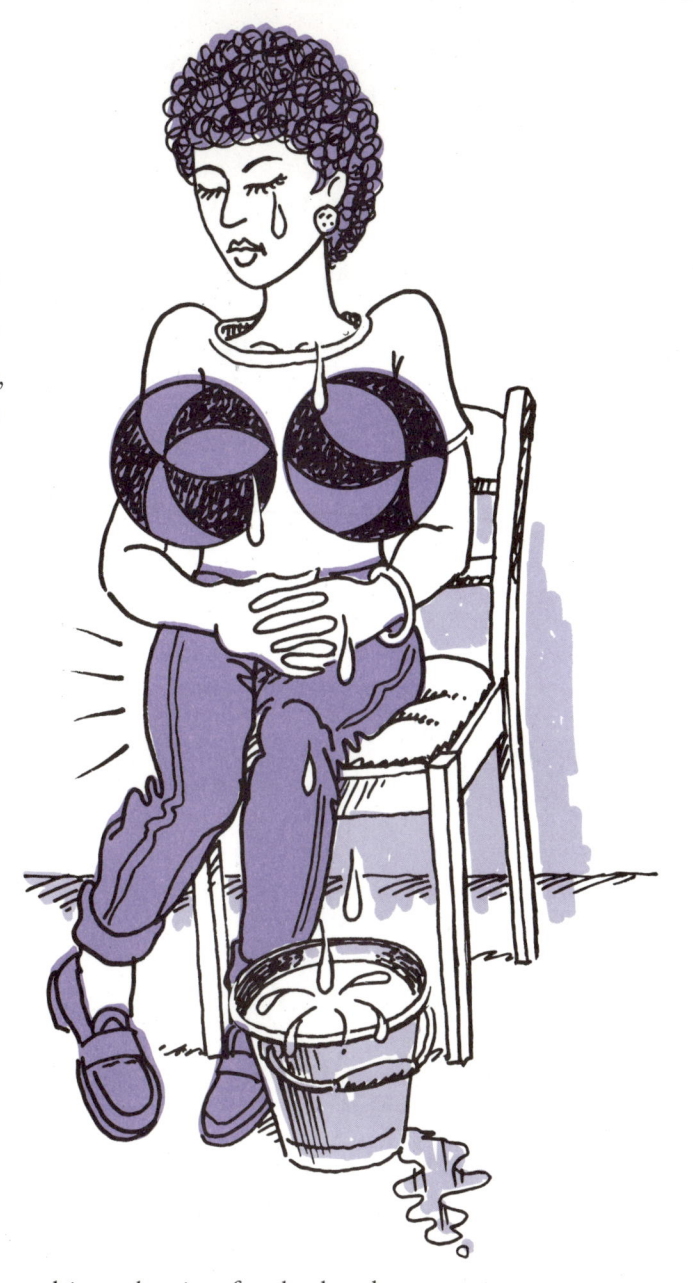

The problem with baby's temperature control is not that

The problem with baby's temperature control is not that they need more insulation, but that they cannot compensate for rapid changes

35

EARLY DAYS

It's not uncommon for babies to lose weight in the first few days

they need more insulation than older people but that they cannot compensate for rapid changes. If we are outside in thin clothes and a cold change comes through, our bodies compensate for that change by shivering and closing down our skin blood flow, retaining the warmth of the core of our bodies. Small babies are not able to compensate as efficiently, so care must be taken to dress the baby appropriately for the current environment and if the temperature changes, to respond accordingly.

Be very careful about exposing your baby to direct sunlight, especially within the first week of life. As their bodies are relatively fluid-deficient in this time, direct sunlight can cause a rapid rise in body temperature and this can be very harmful. Avoid sun kicks until he is a few weeks older and even then it is wise to take special care.

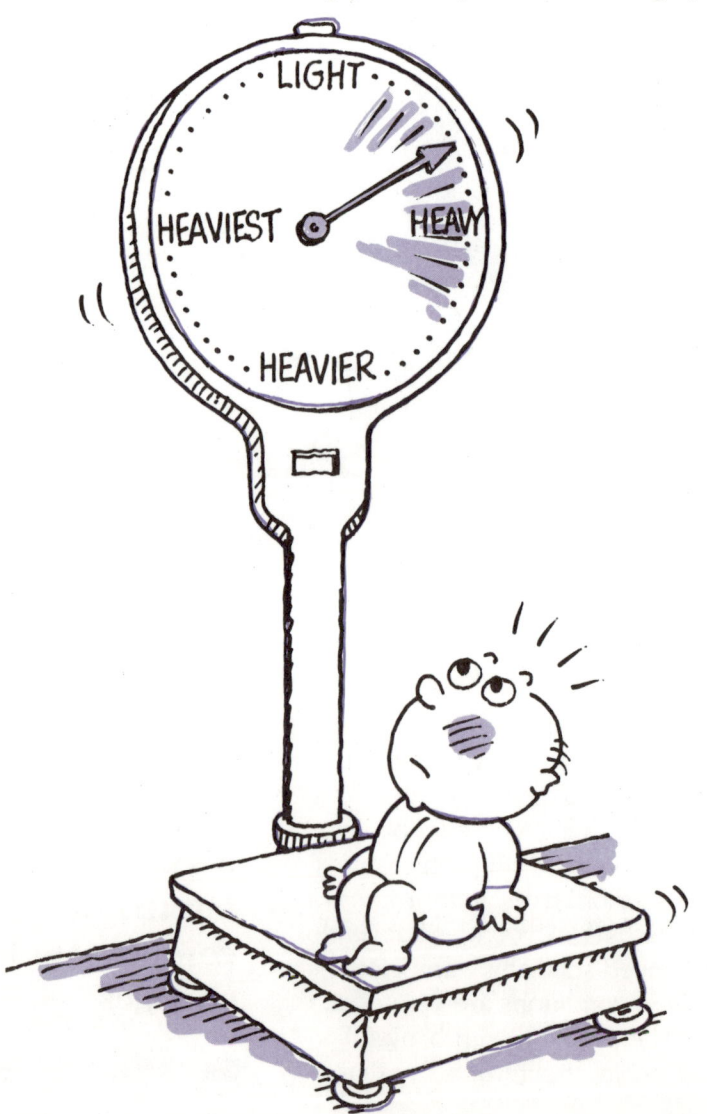

WEIGHT LOSS

When babies are in the womb they are, in effect, marine animals, floating in a primordial sea. When they are born, their bodies are relatively waterlogged and they need to get rid of all that extra water. Nature has arranged this in a very clever way. Firstly, your milk does not come in for a couple of days so the baby does not drink very much. This allows him to get rid of some of his water load. Secondly, he passes urine at a normal rate and therefore loses weight. This is absolutely normal. Many babies will lose up to ten per cent of their body weight (that is 350 g or 12 oz in a normal-sized baby). And this is another reason why babies are relatively uninterested in feeding in the first couple of days. Nature tells them that it's not necessary.

FAT NECROSIS

Some babies develop rubbery lumps under the skin after a few days, usually along the line of the jaw or the cheekbone. This is due to the fat cells in the skin rupturing during delivery. This releases free fat in the skin which sets up an inflammatory reaction. It's quite harmless and the lumps will disappear in a couple of weeks.

EARLY DAYS

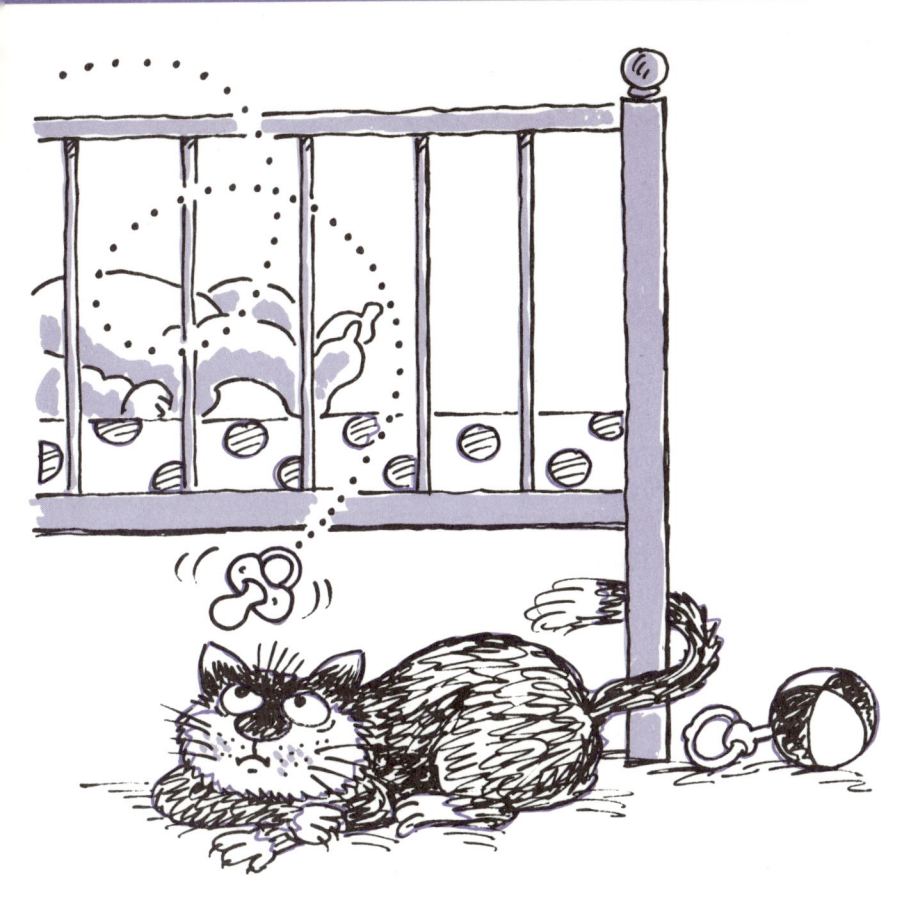

DUMMIES AND THUMB-SUCKING

If a baby wants to suck, he should be allowed to do so. If you don't give him a dummy, he will probably find his fingers or his thumb. All the bad reports about dummies are untrue. However a 'dormel', a miniature bottle filled with sugary drink, dissolves teeth and should never be used. The thumb is probably more convenient than the dummy and tends not to fall on the floor out of reach. Some parents reject dummies because of the appearance, others prefer their babies to have dummies because at some time in the future they can be thrown away (the dummies, that is!). The baby is sucking his thumb or dummy for very good reasons – it calms him, helps him sleep and comforts him. His parents' opinions of the aesthetic aspects don't interest him, and they should mind their own business.

Dummies don't cause disease, and thumbs won't make his teeth stick out and cost you a fortune in orthodontics. Neither will his thumb shrink. For everyone's peace of mind, allow your baby to make up his own mind about whether or not he wishes to suck and, if so, what.

UMBILICAL HERNIA

Some babies develop a swelling under the umbilicus that gets larger when they yell or tense up their tummy. If you squeeze it, it may gurgle and the contents disappear back into the abdomen. This is the one hernia in the body you can completely ignore. It never causes problems, doesn't ever burst, never strangulates and doesn't require surgery. It is just a small gap in the muscle layer of the abdominal wall and is composed of a very strong membrane. It will disappear gradually and in the vast majority of babies is completely gone before the child reaches the age of five, and usually long before that.

UMBILICAL CLEANING

The umbilical cord is usually not mother's favourite part of her baby. Most will touch it only reluctantly and fear that any handling will cause it to start bleeding or will hurt the baby in some way.
Facts:
• The cord has no pain fibres and cutting the cord didn't hurt the baby either.
• The cord is very tough.
• Within an hour of delivery, the arteries are in spasm and bleeding is most unlikely and, as long as the cord remains uninfected, important bleeding is impossible after the first day. Spots of blood from the cord are not a problem.

The cord is cleaned at regular intervals because germs grow readily on its surface and especially in the gutter between the cord and the skin. To clean it, use diluted methylated spirits, and while doing so, gently pull on the cord to get down into the gutter. If your baby cries while this procedure is being done, it is not because it is painful but because the methylated spirits is cold to his skin. If the cord gets smelly, clean it more frequently. If the skin around the umbilicus becomes red, it may be developing an infection so tell your paediatrician or midwife.

37

EARLY DAYS

Usually on the second or third day most babies' skin starts to go a little yellow in colour. This is jaundice. As the days go on this colour may deepen and cause the whites of the eyes to become yellow also.

Jaundice is caused by a substance called bilirubin, the breakdown product of the red pigment in blood

JAUNDICE

This infantile jaundice has no relationship to the jaundice in older children and adults, which is associated with illnesses, especially of the liver. The baby's jaundice is part of the normal process of the baby adapting to life outside his mother's womb.

Jaundice is caused by a substance called bilirubin, which is the breakdown product of haemoglobin, the red pigment in blood. Every day one per cent of the red blood cells in the body is being broken down and this produces bilirubin. While the baby is in the womb this bilirubin is passed across the placenta and processed by mother's liver in order that it can be excreted. The fetus's liver needs to do very little of this work. Once the baby has been born his liver has to 'learn' how to process the bilirubin for itself. This takes a few days and up until that time, the jaundice level of the baby will rise steadily. In most babies it never rises to a high level and nothing need be done about it.

However, in some babies the level may continue to rise higher than average. In *very* high quantities, circulating bilirubin can be dangerous to a baby. It is therefore a good idea to make sure that the jaundice reaches nowhere near such levels. This is done by monitoring the blood bilirubin level, once or twice a day, and if the level is found to be rising quickly or to moderate levels, we start treatment. It must be emphasised, however, that the safety margin is very large and while the baby is under such care, there is no danger at all to his health.

Phototherapy

The level of jaundice in the baby can be controlled using phototherapy. This is a simple procedure, where the naked baby is exposed to ordinary fluorescent light. The bilirubin absorbs the energy from the light and this energy breaks the bilirubin down so that it can be easily excreted. We use the phototherapy as a holding measure until the baby's liver is able to handle the bilirubin for itself. While the baby is under phototherapy, pads are put over his eyes, to stop him being dazzled and help him sleep. These pads do have a tendency to slip off and they should be gently replaced.

When the baby first goes under the lights, his temperature will be taken occasionally to make sure that he doesn't get

EARLY DAYS

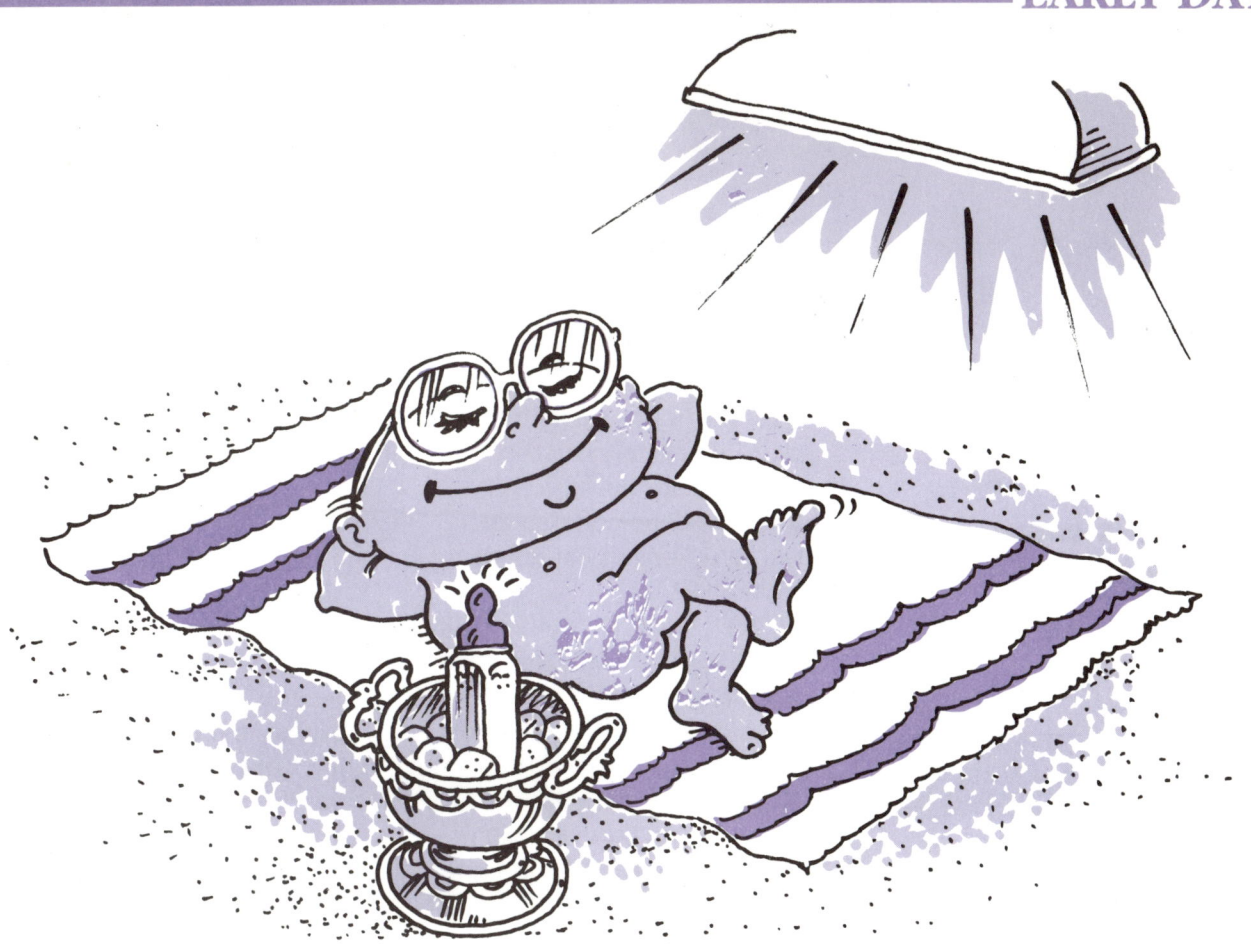

cold. He is fed as normal. Some jaundiced babies, however, are a bit sleepy and are rather lazy on the breast. Under these circumstances, it may be advisable to express your milk and give it to the baby in a bottle, or, unusually, to give baby some formula if feeding is not established. Once the baby's jaundice level starts to come down he usually wakes promptly and feeds much better, so this is just another holding procedure and does not mean that the bottle needs to be continued.

As the jaundice is broken down by the light, the breakdown products are passed out in the stool. These tend to make the stool rather more loose and frequent than before. Also, you may notice it becomes more greenish in colour. These changes merely demonstrate that the phototherapy is doing its job and the jaundice is being eliminated from the body.

Occasionally, some babies (not being used to sunbathing) tend to cry for the first few hours under the lights. This phase will quickly pass as the baby quickly adjusts to his new circumstances.

Prolonged jaundice

The jaundice level starts to come down from about day five onwards, with or without the lights. It then usually drops rapidly over the next few days and unless it looks like it's increasing (a rare happening) it should be ignored. However, it is not unusual for the jaundice, though paler, to remain for some weeks and you can get pretty sick of your friends commenting on your lemon-yellow baby! Such babies are almost invariably breastfed. It seems that some substance in the milk stops the baby's liver completely eliminating the jaundice. It never does any harm at all and if you wait it will slowly fade and disappear. If you're tired of your friends' amusing references to the little lemon, you could try stopping breastfeeding for forty-eight hours. During this time, feed the baby formula and express your breasts to keep up your milk flow. Freeze the milk for the baby-sitter to use later. This might hasten the disappearance of the jaundice but it doesn't always work.

BREAST IS BEST

Breast is best! There's no argument about it. It's cheap and it's perfect for the baby in every way.

Getting started with breastfeeding is not necessarily easy. In humans it is not instinctive and needs to be taught

BREASTFEEDING

Breastfeeding virtually immunises him against bacterial gastroenteritis and there is a lower incidence of respiratory tract infections in babies who are breastfed.

Breast milk is always readily available at the right temperature and best of all, breastfeeding is enjoyable. Having your baby sucking on your breast can release wonderful pleasure-producing hormones which tranquillise and reward you for doing it.

However, it is much better if you *want* to breastfeed your baby for reasons other than that you think it's good for him. Self-sacrifice is something all children expect from their mothers, but not in this instance.

Babies prefer their mothers to feed them in the way that makes her happier, more relaxed and less tired. If breastfeeding does that, and for most it will, go for it; but if you feel that the bottle is the way for you, go for that.

Getting started with breastfeeding is not necessarily easy. It is a strange phenomenon that in the primate (that is, higher mammals such as apes) breastfeeding is not an instinctive ability, it needs to be taught. In chimpanzee troupes the older females teach the younger ones how to do it. This is illustrated by zoo experience with gorillas. Because there are usually only a few in any zoo, if a female has a baby there is usually no experienced female to teach her how to feed it. To overcome this, techniques such as allowing the gorilla to watch humans breastfeed, or videotapes of gorillas feeding their young, have been used, but often with only limited success.

Maternity hospitals have lots of experienced staff to help you get started – make sure you make use of this vital resource.

Attaching the baby to the breast

Many babies, if allowed to do so, will suck on the nipple like a bottle teat. This is the wrong technique, producing no colostrum for him and soreness (and

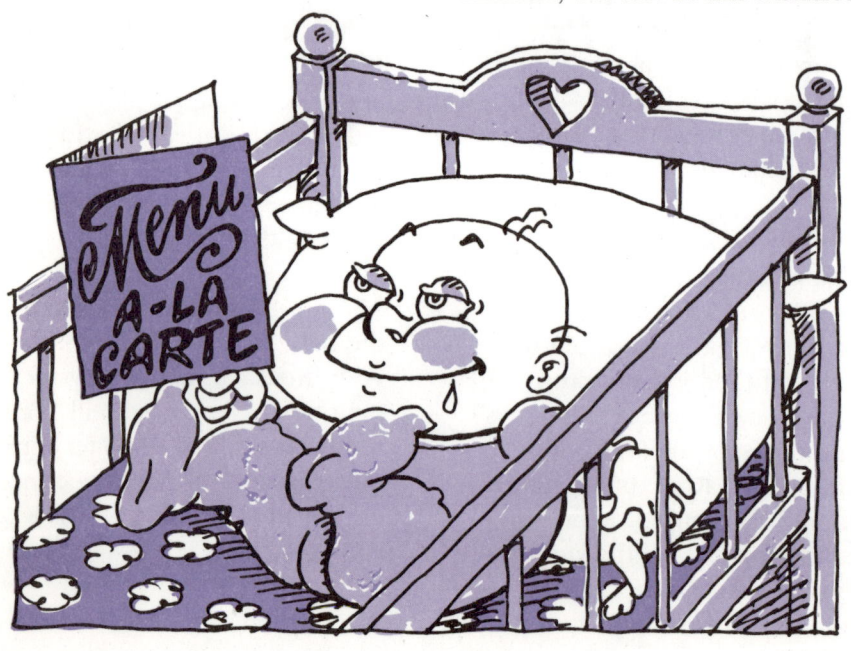

BREAST IS BEST

even blistering) of the nipple for you. Getting your baby attached properly is CRITICAL to breastfeeding, so get the best help you can for the early feeds.

Your baby should be presented with the breast, ideally before he is howling and tense, so you and he are as relaxed as possible. Make sure you are comfortable, sitting or lying on your side. Unwrap the baby so that you can both enjoy the skin contact – if it's a cool day put a blanket over both of you. Gently talk to him and let his lips stroke your nipple and he should respond by opening his mouth wide and 'rooting' for it. The idea then is to get the whole of the nipple into his mouth so he can hold it by suction up against the back of his palate. This will draw much of the areola (the pigmented area around the nipple) into his mouth, so that there may be only a rim of it outside his mouth above and none below. This immobilises the breast and allows him to squeeze the milk ducts which lie under the areola. He does this by:

- chomping on that area with jaw action (you can see the muscles right out to his ears move as he does it) – if he sucks in his cheeks he's not on properly; and
- a rolling action with his tongue, from the front of his mouth to the back.

Both of these cause the colostrum or milk to squirt out of the breast into his throat to be swallowed. The process usually has some help from the 'let-down' reflex.

The nipple is only used to immobilise the breast in the

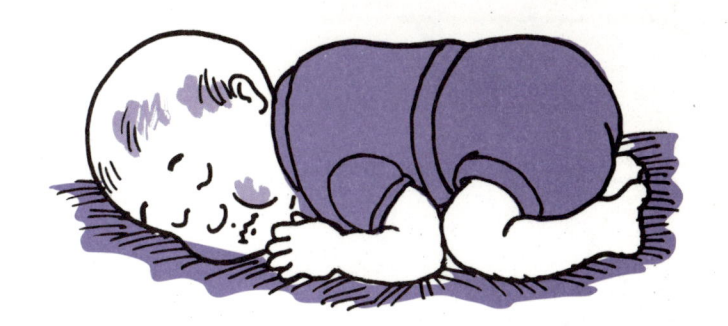

SEVEN STEPS TO SUCCESSFUL BREASTFEEDING

1 Start as early as possible, hopefully in the first couple of hours and certainly within the first twelve.

2 Make sure an experienced midwife teaches you how to attach your baby to the breast properly from the beginning.

3 Demand feed the baby right from the start.

4 Feed the baby for as long as he wants to at every feed – within reason. If the feeds are taking longer than thirty minutes after the milk has come in, perhaps he's not attached well or his positioning is wrong so he finds it difficult to swallow.

5 If your nipples get sore, it's a warning that something needs adjusting, either the baby's attachment to the breast or his position. It's NOT that he's sucking too long or that he's sucking too vigorously.

6 Don't miss the night feeds. It's likely they boost your milk supply even more than daytime feeds. Feeding is also tranquillising and may help you sleep better.

7 Don't wash your nipples other than in normal hygiene. The nipple produces substances that attract your baby and help him attach to the breast. Don't use creams, lotions, potions or that magic ointment that the old lady round the corner says will stop nipple soreness. Change breast pads often and try to spend a little time with your breasts uncovered. Studies show that the best thing for your nipples, sore or otherwise, is nothing at all.

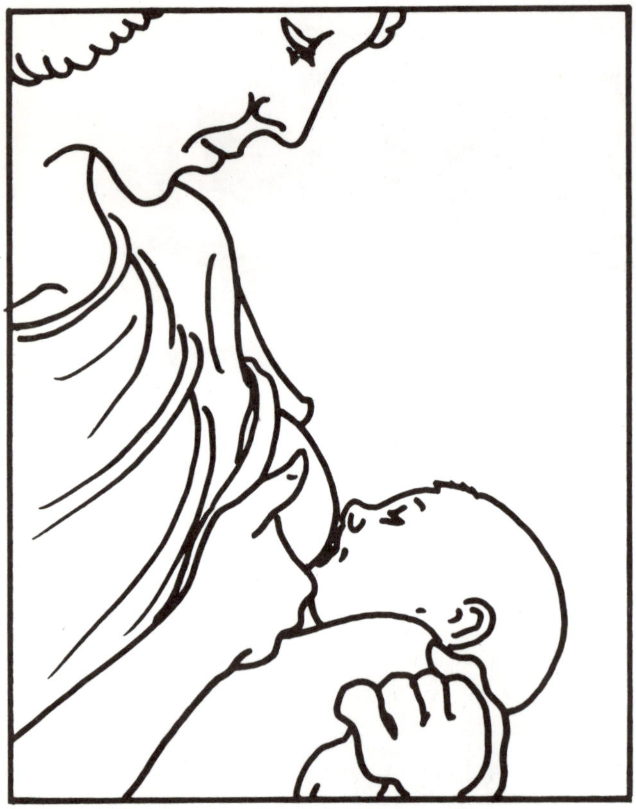

BREAST IS BEST

Finding a comfortable feeding posture is most important

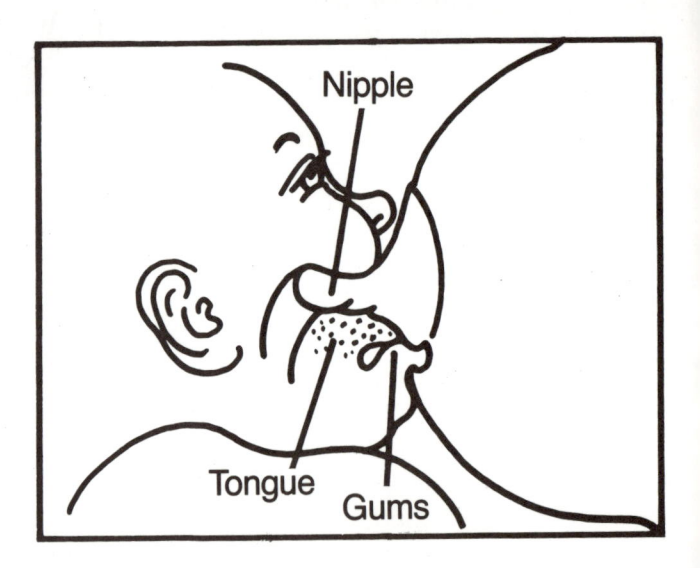

This is the appearance of correct attachment. Note that the nipple is pointed slightly towards the roof of the mouth

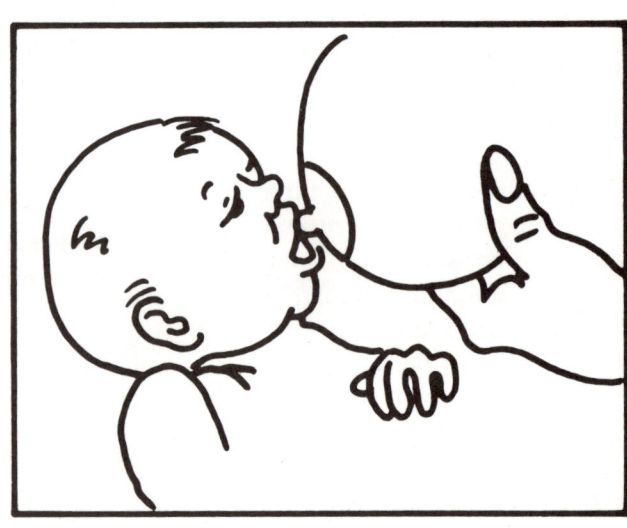

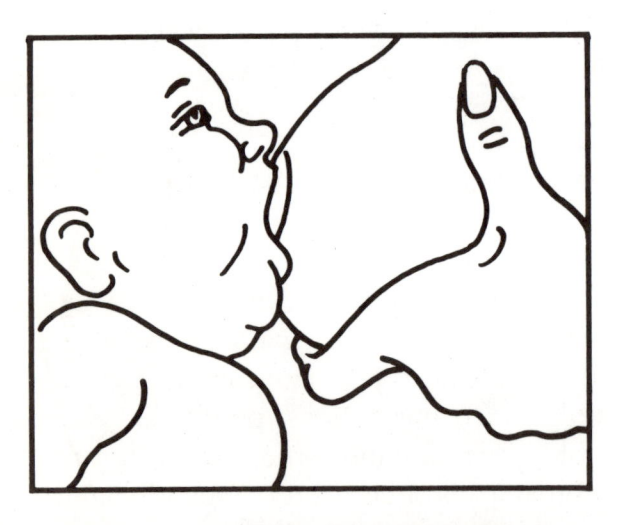

The nipple is immobilised by suction against the palate, while the jaws chomp and the tongue rolls from the front to the back of the mouth

Let the baby's lips stroke the nipple and he should respond by opening his mouth wide and 'rooting' for it

BREAST IS BEST

mouth. There is no rubbing of the skin and no reason for soreness to develop if the attachment is right.

Positioning the baby
- Make sure you are both comfortable and relaxed.
- Let the breast fall into the baby's mouth naturally, don't PUT it there.
- The baby's head shouldn't be too flexed or extended – you try swallowing with your neck stretched or scrunched up!
- If you are having to press the breast to avoid it obstructing his nose, change his position so the nipple points more towards the roof of his mouth.
- Supporting the baby on your arm, with his body across the front of yours, or under your arm are common positions, as is lying down with both of you on your side.

The let-down reflex
The milk ducts that collect the milk produced in the breast lie behind the nipple, under the areola and adjacent breast tissue. They have muscle fibres in their walls and, under the action of the hormone oxytocin (the same hormone that contracts your uterus), they contract and eject their milk. This explains the 'after-pains' you get in your uterus, especially when you feed the baby, and why feeding the baby soon after delivery is so good to help the uterus contract.

A mother can often feel this reflex as a tingle at the beginning of a feed. Sometimes a hungry cry from her baby is enough on its own to initiate the let-down reflex.

First days
Many babies in the first two or three days are sleepy and not wildly enthusiastic about feeding. It's not really surprising as there is no more than a dribble of colostrum for them when they wake and, being sensible people, they do only what is rewarding. Take the opportunity to get some rest, because when your milk comes in a little light will come on in your baby's head, and your life will not be the same again!

Colostrum
Sometimes even before you have had your baby but in increasing quantities after, the breast produces colostrum. This

Many babies in the first few days are sleepy and not wildly enthusiastic about feeding

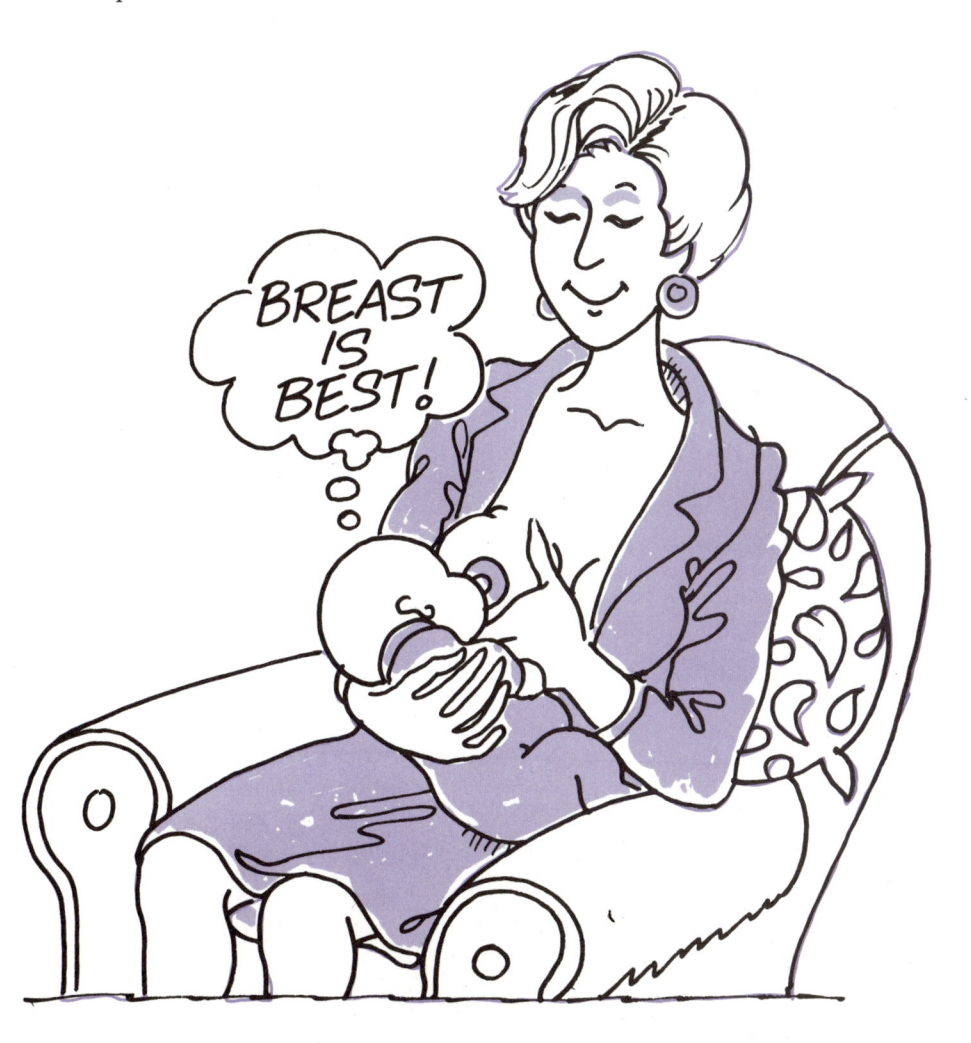

BREAST IS BEST

> **You should feed your baby as long as he likes, as long as it is less than about half an hour**

Breast milk

Breast milk is always of top quality. You never need have any doubt about that. Its normal appearance is opalescent and pearly, rather than white and although it may look more watery than formula, do not be deceived. If the baby is not thriving after a week or so, the only question is the quantity being produced, not its quality.

There are only two factors that will increase your breast milk flow – the main one is rest and the other is more sucking, stimulation and emptying of the breast. If you get overtired it is likely your milk supply will suffer. An afternoon nap might be essential for you to maintain your milk flow.

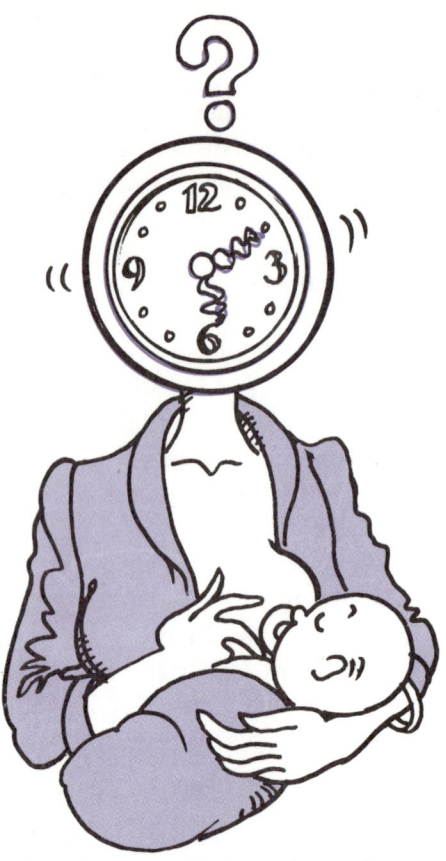

is a clear to yellow-coloured fluid, which is full of antibodies and immunity promoting cells. These substances line the baby's bowel and set up the start of immunity against gastroenteritis. It is certainly good for the baby, but it is not too much of a problem if the baby misses out on it for any reason. The bowel will catch up when the breast milk is available.

Milk 'coming in'

The milk 'comes in' at about two and a half days and following that, especially for the next twenty-four hours, the baby demands much more often, sometimes one or two hourly. This can really wear you out, but have no fear. Your baby will settle down as he gets used to the milk and he will feed for longer periods of time less frequently.

How long should feeding my baby take?

You should feed your baby for as long as he likes, as long as it is less than about half an hour, unless you don't mind being used as a dummy and you both enjoy it. Ideally he should stay on the first breast until he stops sucking and falls off. It is not necessary to time him so he gets both breasts equally each feed. Actually towards the end of a feed the milk is richer in fat (hence relatively more calories) so he finds it more satisfying. If he wants more then offer the other breast, but if he's not interested – don't. Then next feed, start with the other breast to even things up.

Not enough milk

The more the breast is sucked and the more milk is withdrawn from it, the more milk there will be produced. It is a very neat

BREAST IS BEST

feed-back mechanism (no pun intended!). As for substances you can take to increase your milk flow (called lactogogues), other than a drug called meta-clopramide which has a small effect in some mothers and no effect in others, no-one has ever shown that anything makes any difference – not stout, brewer's yeast, herbs or extra fluids. So don't waste the time you could spend resting. If there were some effective lactogogues available you can be sure that the dairy farmers would know about it – and they have no magic answers either.

Too much milk

When the milk first comes in, very commonly the breasts become engorged – it could be called the 'beach ball syndrome'. Luckily, this only lasts twelve to twenty-four hours and is usually relieved by a warm shower, a couple of paracetamol tablets and gentle expression of a little of the milk to take the tension out of the breast. If the breasts are very tight, the baby sometimes cannot attach properly and a little hand expression of milk before the feed can help soften them. Do not attempt to empty the breast as it will merely fill up again. Do not use mechanical milk expressers, only the hand ones.

Sore nipples

Luckily, the nipples have a very high blood flow and if the attachment to the breast is corrected (sorry to go on about this so much but you're probably getting the message that it is crucial) they will heal rapidly. If you have cracked or blistered nipples it is a good idea to gently express that breast and feed the baby only on the other side. Then start again on that breast after twenty-four hours. Only in extreme cases is gentle hand expression and feeding the baby breast milk from a bottle necessary. Luckily, nipples heal quickly, so hang in there.

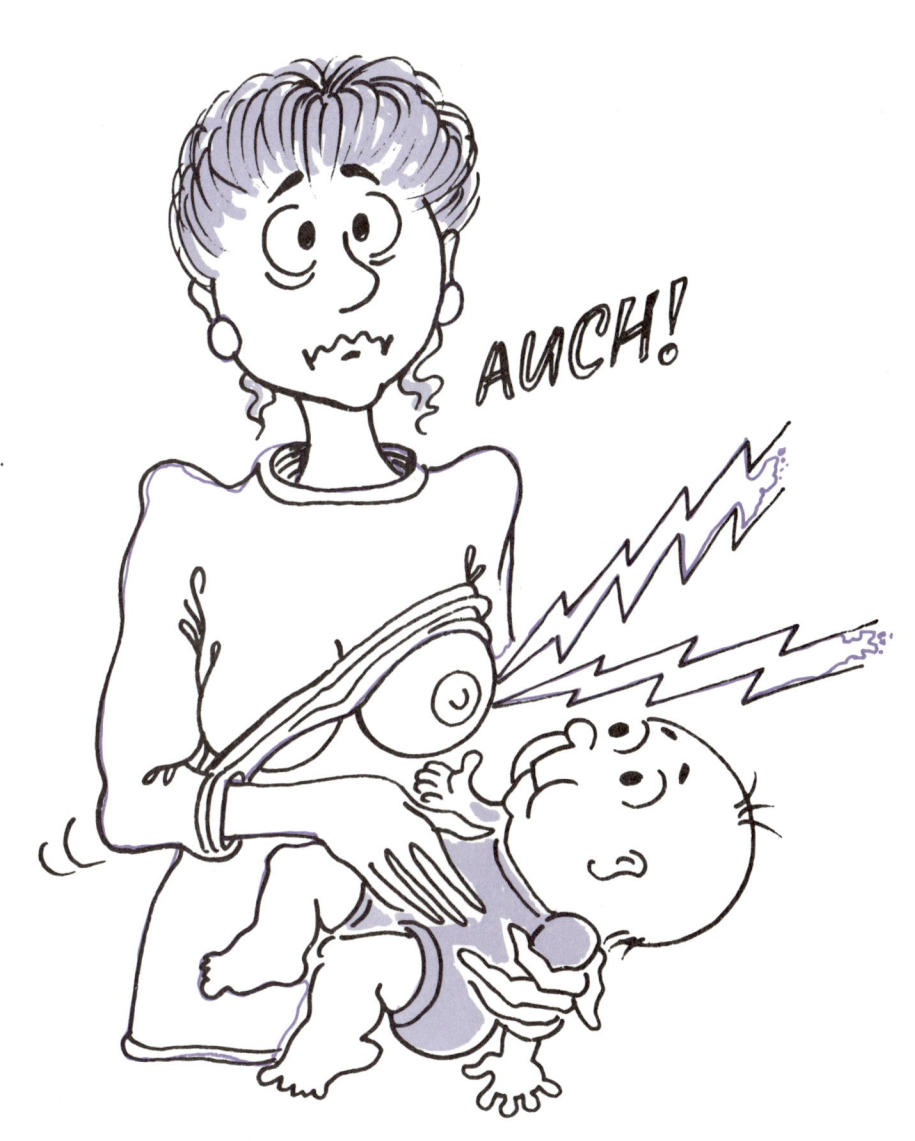

BREAST IS BEST

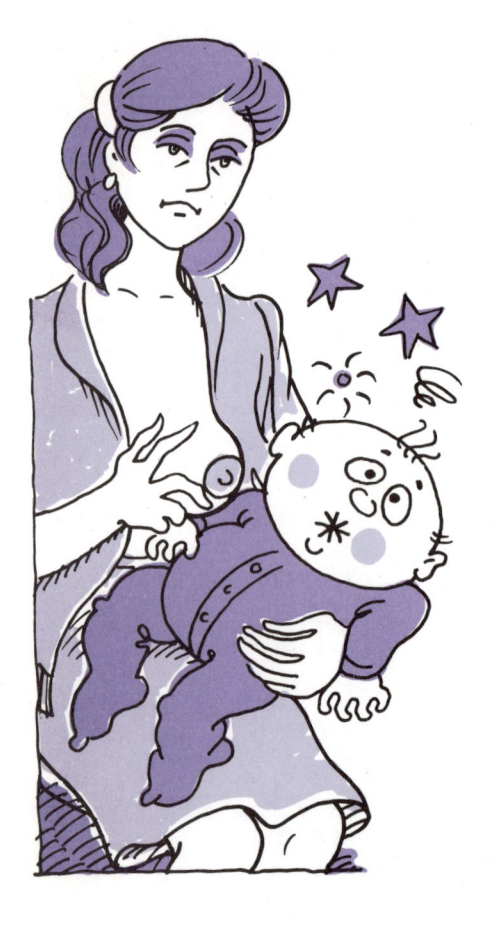

In summary

Except for the technique of attachment and positioning, your baby needs very little supervision regarding his feeding. Nature is not so dumb that we need three hands, a stopwatch, electronic scales and tubes of nipple cream in order to successfully feed our babies. The correct phrase to describe the process is 'baby-led' feeding. We know from detailed research that babies will provide themselves with the right amount of calories if offered the breast (and often only one is necessary) and allowed to direct when to stop and when to switch breasts. So let your baby drive – he knows the way to go.

Water feeds

It is most unusual for your baby to become dehydrated, so he should not be offered water feeds. There is never an indication for glucose and water as this will just make your baby vomit and will offer him very little nourishment. Your baby is very well designed to cope with barely a dribble of feed for two or three days or even longer, so he will come to no harm if you both patiently await the arrival of breast milk.

Drugs in breast milk

Most mothers who are on medication are very concerned that the drug might be passed through to the baby in the breast milk. Happily there are very few drugs which get into breast milk in quantities that have any effect on the baby. So most common antibiotics; antihistamines; antidepressants (even lithium); antihypertensives; tranquillisers; analgesics (aspirin, paracetamol and codeine); laxatives; and drugs that act on the heart, are harmless.

If you are taking anticonvulsants, such as phenobarbitone or phenytoin, you can still breastfeed but your doctor will make sure that the dosage is correct for you both.

The list would not be complete, however, if we left off alcohol, which is fine as long as you don't overdose, and nico-

---

BREASTFEEDING – BEWARE!

These drugs can be secreted in the milk in amounts that affect the baby.

- Tetracycline
- Anti-cancer drugs (antimetabolites or cytotoxics)
- Long-acting radioisotopes (if you have special X-ray examinations tell the doctor you're breastfeeding)
- Anti-thyroid drugs and iodides
- Bromide
- Oral hypoglycaemic agents (for diabetes)
- Some sex hormones (don't take high-dose oral contraceptives)
- Some cortisones (but prednisone is OK)
- Some anti-rheumatism drugs (gold salts, indomethacin or phenylbutazone)
- Anti migraine drugs containing ergot
- Heroin

BREAST IS BEST

tine from cigarette smoke, which isn't fine at all. In fact one of the breakdown products of nicotine is found in large quantities in the milk and in the urine of the babies of smoking mothers. Do your little newcomer and yourself a big favour, and quit.

If you are to be prescribed a drug, you should, of course, tell the doctor you are breastfeeding, just to be on the safe side.

BOTTLE-FEEDING

If you want to bottle-feed your baby, do so. The main advantage of breastfeeding is that it is easier. If that is not the case in your life, then don't let anybody make you feel guilty about it. Babies prefer their mothers to be well rested and happy than to be breastfed at any cost. An advantage of bottle-feeding is that dad and other people can help out which, particularly if you are a working mother, is very helpful.

The formulas available today are nutritionally very similar to breast milk and using them, babies will thrive and grow at just the same rate. They are derived from cow's milk or use vegetable protein from the soya bean. There are many different formulas available and all are now 'humanised', meaning they contain close to the same amount of protein, carbohydrate, fat and minerals as breast milk. In addition, many also contain extra vitamins and iron in recommended dosages. In choosing a formula, get the one that is easiest for you to obtain and stick to it. Don't listen too hard to other mothers' stories or you'll be chopping and changing every time junior vomits. None of the major formulas make babies vomit (but they all taste awful to adults). Most of them are available in concentrated liquid or powdered form, the former being marginally easier to make up, but rather more expensive.

If you want to bottle-feed your baby, and it suits your lifestyle, then go ahead

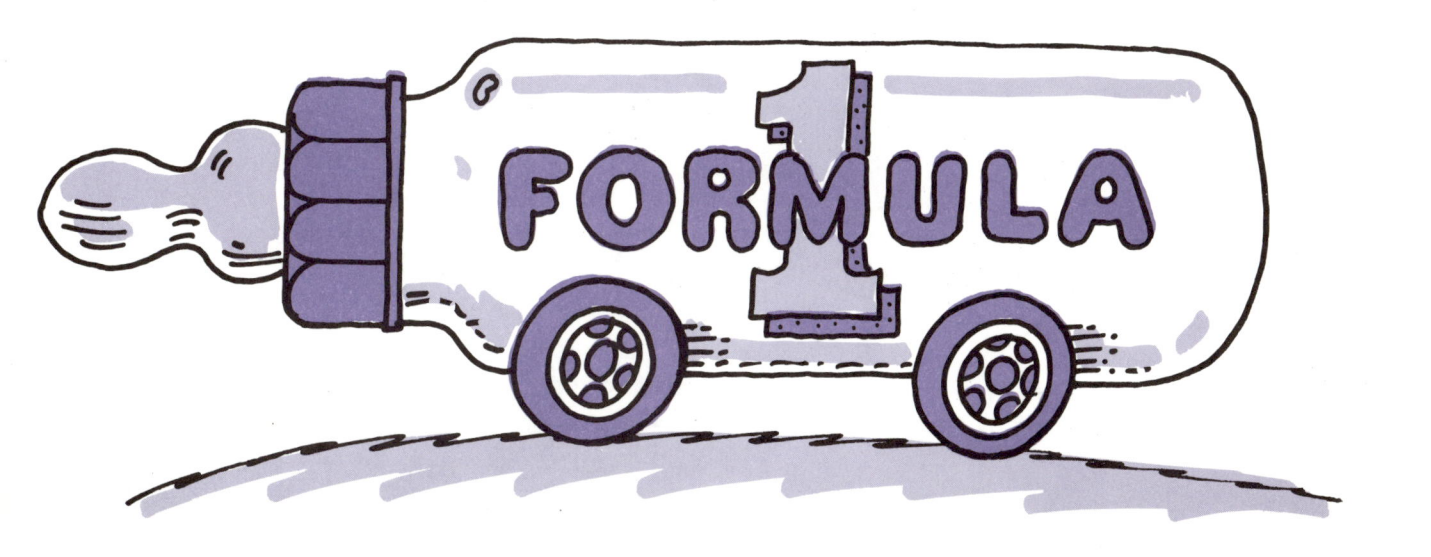

47

BREAST IS BEST

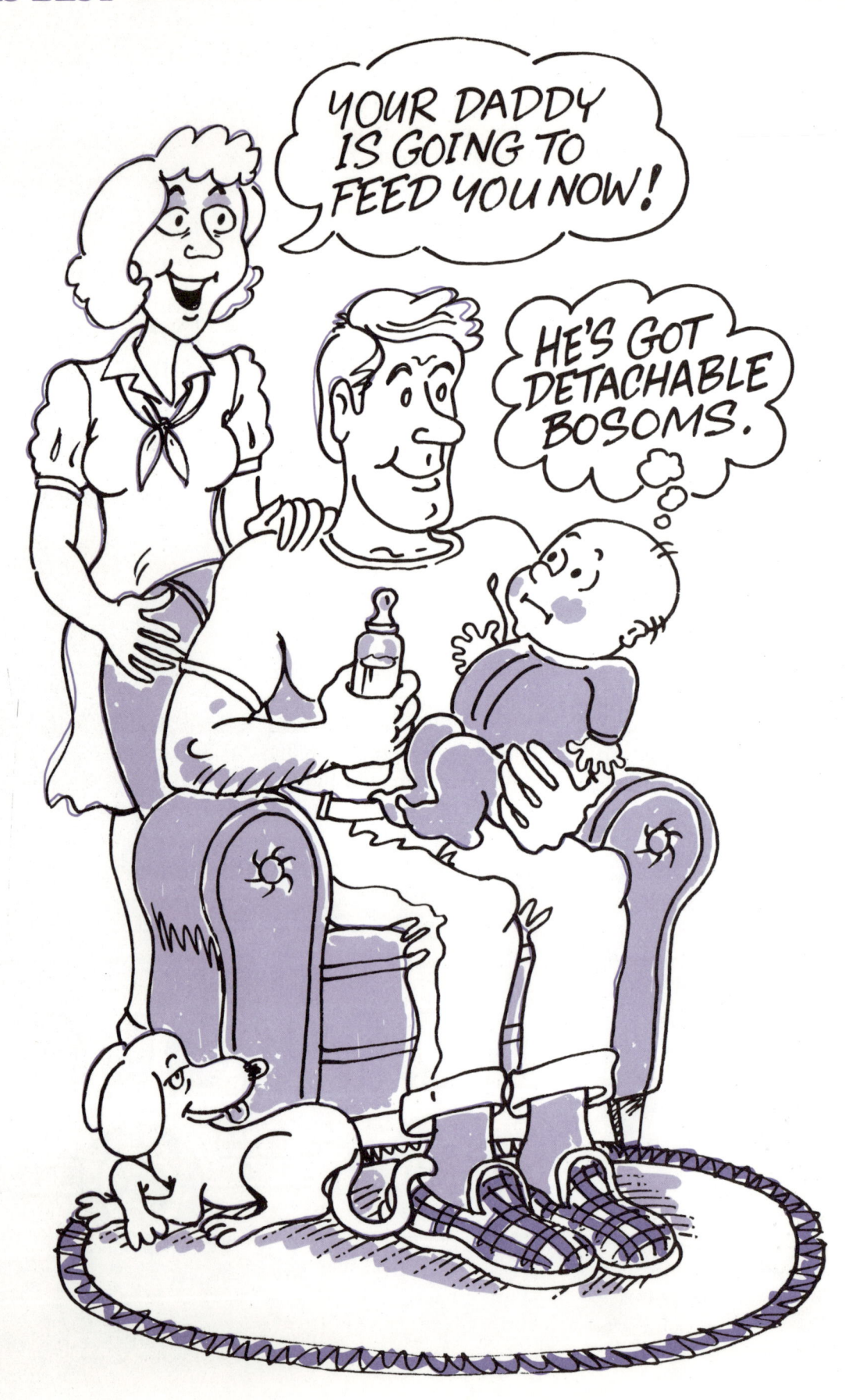

BREAST IS BEST

Using formula, it is very important to observe cleanliness of hands and sterility of bottle and teat. Set aside a can-opener and knife (for smoothing off the scoops of powder) just for making up the formula and prepare a whole twenty-four hours' supply in one go, keeping the made up formula in the refrigerator. Make up rather more than you calculate he actually needs for the day. Boil the water for the formula for a full ten minutes, then let it become lukewarm before pouring it into a sterile jug (or his bottle) and adding **level** scoops of formula powder. Never add any more powder than is recommended in the directions on the tin, as the exact concentration of powder in the water is critical.

When you feed him his bottle, treat it as you would a breastfeed. Give him all your attention and, if you like, your skin contact. He would enjoy it if you took your blouse off and cuddled him during a feed, and you probably would too. You needn't actually warm his formula as babies will take it cold just as well, but that's up to you.

How much you feed him is up to him. He should be demand fed when he's hungry, and not by the clock. At the end of the feed if there is something left in the bottle and he's not sucking anymore, he's had enough. **On average** (note the emphasis) a baby takes about 160 mL per kilo of his body weight a day, but that's an average baby on an average day. Don't insist on exact amounts each feed. Like us, sometimes he'll want more and sometimes less.

When he's finished, rinse the bottle and teat straight away to remove formula before it dries, and always discard formula left over in the bottle from a feed or at the end of twenty-four hours.

Beware of using microwave ovens for warming formula or for thawing frozen breastmilk. They really heat the milk but the bottle still feels cold. Anyway, always check the temperature of the milk by sprinkling a little from the bottle onto the inner part of your wrist.

Remember if you are travelling to a developing country, be very careful of bad water supply or drainage, and make sure reliable refrigeration is available. Your baby is vulnerable to gastroenteritis if he is bottle-fed. Under these circumstances a real effort to breastfeed is very worthwhile.

DOING BOTH

It is usually fairly difficult to both breast and bottle-feed except as a temporary measure, for instance when weaning the baby or trying to build up one's milk supply. Doing both, you get many of the disadvantages of both methods and few of the advantages of either. Formula dilutes the antibodies in breast milk that protect the baby from bacterial gastroenteritis and the convenience of bottle-feeding is lost if you also have to breastfeed. Feeding can also take too long. However there may be some subtle advantages to any amount of breast milk, such as tiny amounts of growth factors, hormones and other substances only half-understood at present. So do both if it suits you both.

The milk formulas available nowadays are nutritionally very similar to breast milk and babies will thrive on them just as well

BREAST IS BEST

Babies are better burpers than we are

LACTOSE INTOLERANCE

Lactose intolerance in the baby who has not suffered a bout of gastroenteritis is most unusual. It is normal for a fully breastfed baby to spill some lactose in his stool. These babies tend to be the ones who produce rather explosive frothy stools fairly frequently. This is not an indication to stop breastfeeding and it will usually pass with time. If, however, your baby is taking a few, say four per day, very large feeds you could attempt to feed him more often. This may give the intestine the lactose more gradually and improve absorption. If, however, he tends to 'snack' and only takes the foremilk from the breast, which is rich in lactose, he might be persuaded to feed for longer on the same breast to get the fat-rich, hindmilk.

In extreme cases of lactose spillage into the stool, a few days on a lactose-free formula is usually enough to correct the situation and then breastfeeding should be reintroduced. But I emphasise, this situation is very unusual.

BURPING

Babies are better burpers than we are. The valve between the stomach and the gullet is extremely inefficient in newborn babies and develops better tone as the months pass. Many babies have a very poor hold on their feed and are very likely to posset or regurgitate parts of it during or after the feed. This is even more likely to occur if the baby is postured head down. Consequently, the idea that a baby can trap an air bubble behind this valve which needs ritualised back pounding to release it, doesn't make a lot of sense. If babies don't burp after they have been fed there are two possibilities.

- The baby didn't swallow any air and there is nothing to burp.
- He will burp it later.

Neither of these possibilities is to be feared. Air bubbles in the bowel do not cause pain or

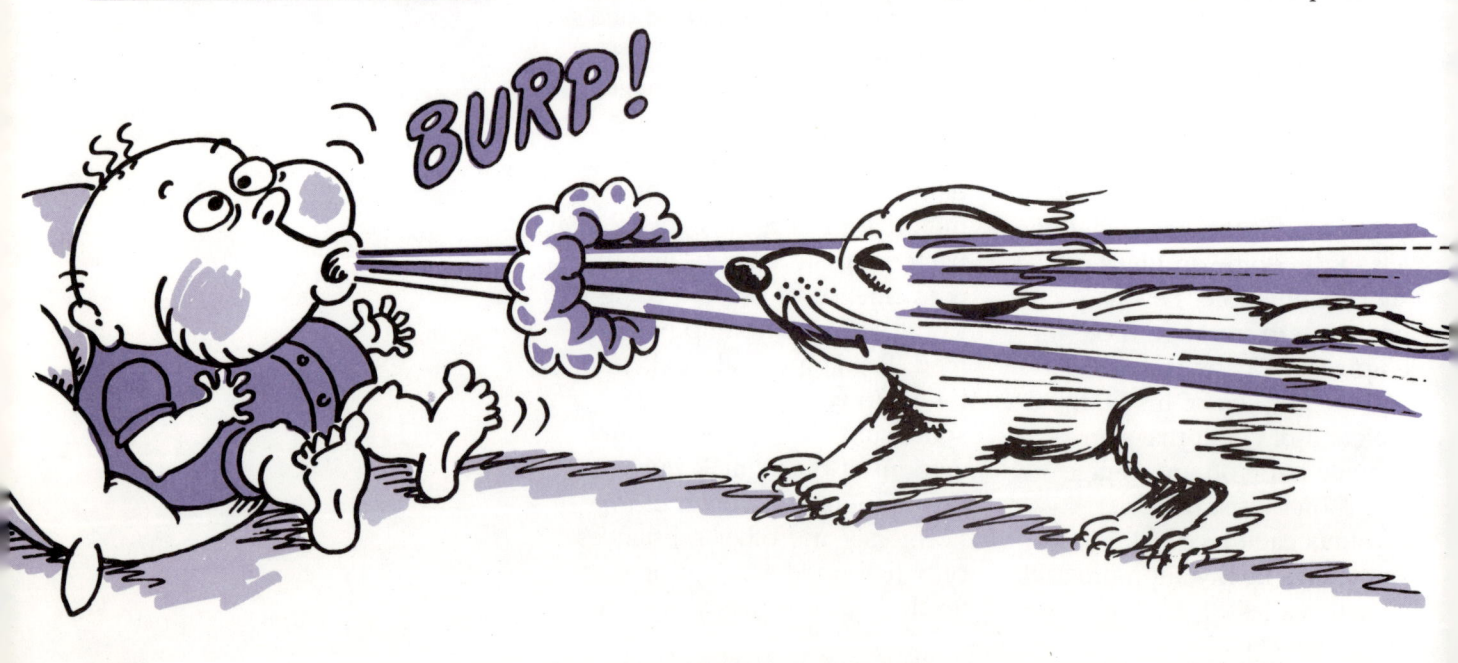

BREAST IS BEST

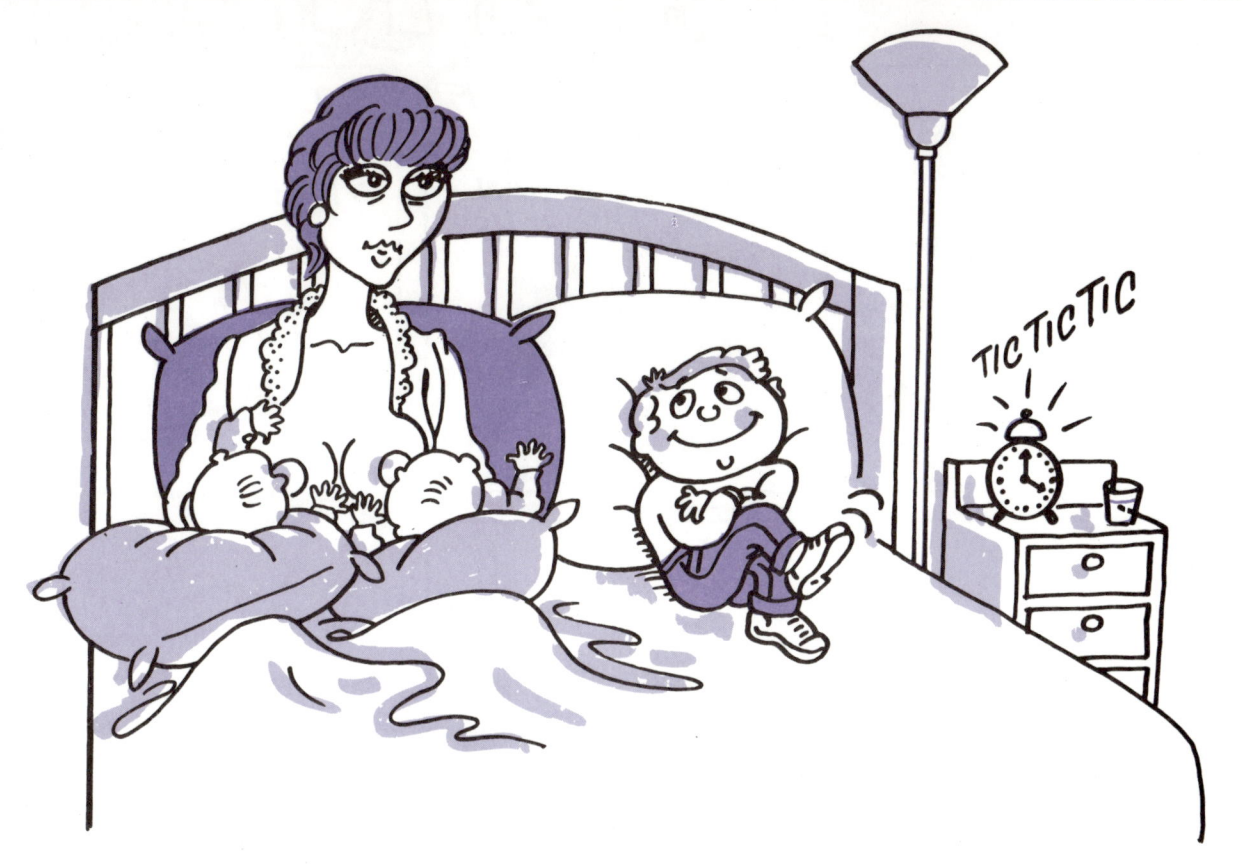

discomfort, distension or spasm. Following a feed all you need to do is to sit the baby up and give him a cuddle and if he wishes to burp, he will. Can you imagine having a satisfying, filling, tranquillising, delightful meal, and then have someone pound you between the shoulder blades before the coffee? Better to let the baby drift off to sleep and put him gently back in his cot (for more on this see the section on 'Colic' on page 70).

TWINS AND MORE

Twins are rather more than twice the work of one. Under these circumstances forget ideology. If one is awake and hungry, wake the other baby and feed them both – either together (the easier method if you've got the technique of attaching one to each breast) or one straight after the other.

Demand feeding is usually too hard and you'll be dead on your feet in a week. Some mothers can feed both babies entirely on the breast and it is definitely worth a try. However, it's a lot of milk to produce, especially in the face of tiredness, so keep an eye on their weight gain and complement with formula if necessary.

VOMITING

The valve between the gullet and the stomach in the newborn baby is extremely weak. If this valve is hanging open as the stomach squeezes to push the milk down into the bowel, the milk is just as likely to be squeezed up and out. This vomiting can even be projectile. X-ray studies of newborn babies show that this possibility occurs in most babies, but it improves rapidly with time. If it occurs

Demand feeding for twins is usually too hard and for triplets, well nigh impossible

often enough to be a worry:
- Sit the baby up after feeds.
- Put him face downwards in his cot in a head-up position. Up to thirty degrees is ideal, but he will tend to slide down the cot unless you put him in a carrying harness with the straps tied to the top of the cot.
- He will probably need topping up right away.

What a pity it is that we use the expression 'being sick' for vomiting. Most babies vomit – rarely is this a sign of sickness.

THE NEW

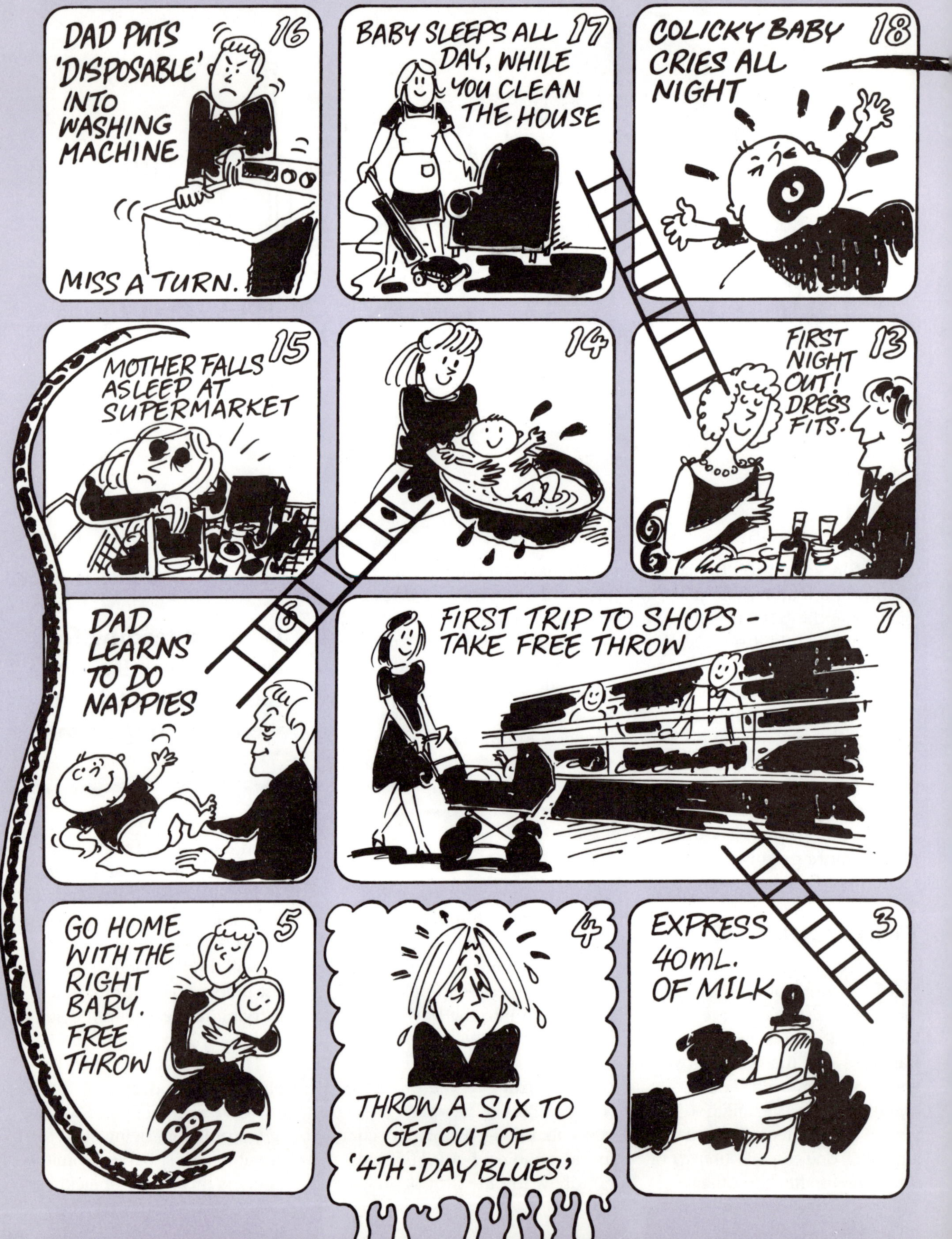
3
EXPRESS 40mL. OF MILK
4
THROW A SIX TO GET OUT OF '4TH-DAY BLUES'
5
GO HOME WITH THE RIGHT BABY. FREE THROW
6
DAD LEARNS TO DO NAPPIES
7
FIRST TRIP TO SHOPS - TAKE FREE THROW
13
FIRST NIGHT OUT! DRESS FITS.
14
15
MOTHER FALLS ASLEEP AT SUPERMARKET
16
DAD PUTS 'DISPOSABLE' INTO WASHING MACHINE
MISS A TURN.
17
BABY SLEEPS ALL DAY, WHILE YOU CLEAN THE HOUSE
18
COLICKY BABY CRIES ALL NIGHT

BABY GAME

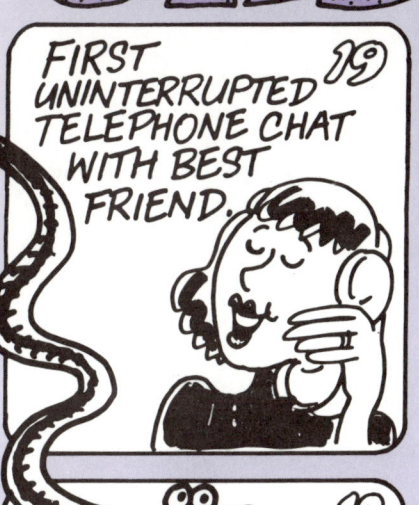

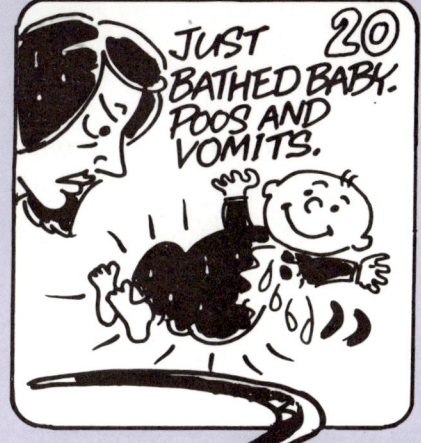

19 FIRST UNINTERRUPTED TELEPHONE CHAT WITH BEST FRIEND.

20 JUST BATHED BABY. POOS AND VOMITS.

FINISH CONGRATULATIONS! YOU HAVE SUCCESSFULLY NEGOTIATED THE FIRST 12 WEEKS OF PARENTHOOD!

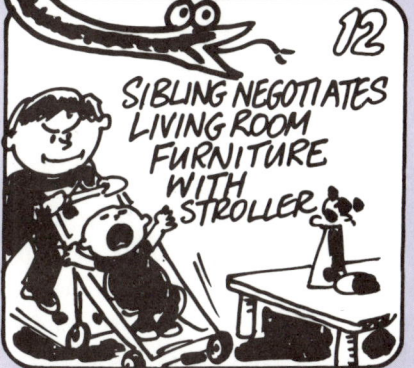

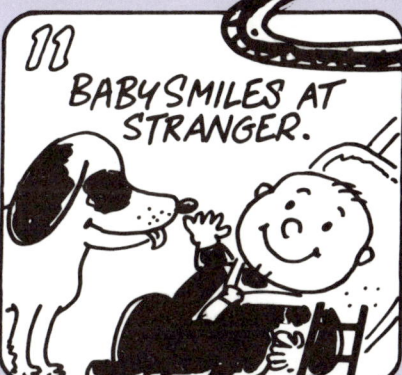

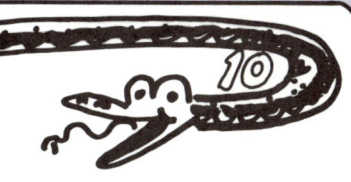

12 SIBLING NEGOTIATES LIVING ROOM FURNITURE WITH STROLLER.

11 BABY SMILES AT STRANGER.

10
a. BABY SMILES AT MOTHER-IN-LAW
b. BABY SLEEPS THROUGH THUNDERSTORM
c. SIBLING FEEDS BABY BOTTLE:

TAKE A FREE TURN.

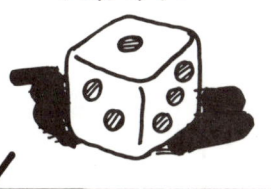

8 FORGOT TO STERILIZE BOTTLES. GO BACK 4 SPACES

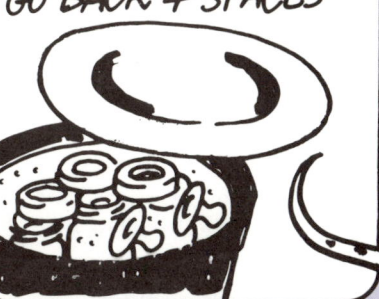

9 BABY SLEEPS 6 HOURS BETWEEN NIGHT FEEDS.

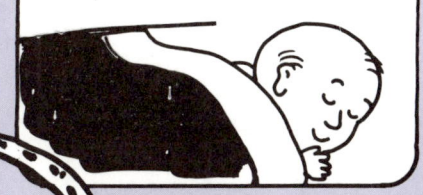

2 FIRST BIG POO. FREE THROW.

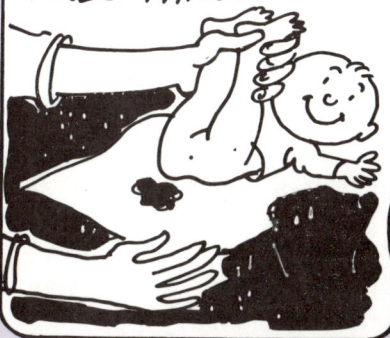

1 MILK COMES IN. BREAST FEED SUCCESSFULLY.

START HERE

YOUR CHILD IS BORN! THROW A SIX TO MOVE.

SETTLING IN

Most first-time mothers choose to have their babies in hospital, although home births are still popular. There are advantages to both alternatives.

GOING HOME

Most first-time mothers can't wait to get home after having their babies. Significantly, most second-time mothers have to be prised out of their hospital bed and sent home, kicking and screaming! There is a lesson here for first-timers. Remember not only does the housework await you, but when your friends visit they now expect to have a cup of tea, wake the baby for a cuddle and usually stay too long.

There are a few things to consider before going home:

1 Your anxiety level about your baby is likely to increase.
2 You will tend to rush around a lot more so that it is likely that you will be more tired and as a result your breast milk will diminish slightly over the first day or two.
3 The combination of these factors is likely to make your baby behave differently for a few days and this can make points 1 and 2 worse.

My advice therefore is:

• Expect a change in your baby's behaviour and accept it. Remember that his behaviour changed from day to day in hospital and will continue to do so at home until a pattern is established.
• Ignore the housework, or get dad to do it, and rest as much as possible.

SIBLINGS

Imagine how it must be. You are two years old and the supreme ruler of your family. One day your parents bring home a baby, a young pretender to your throne, and mummy, your

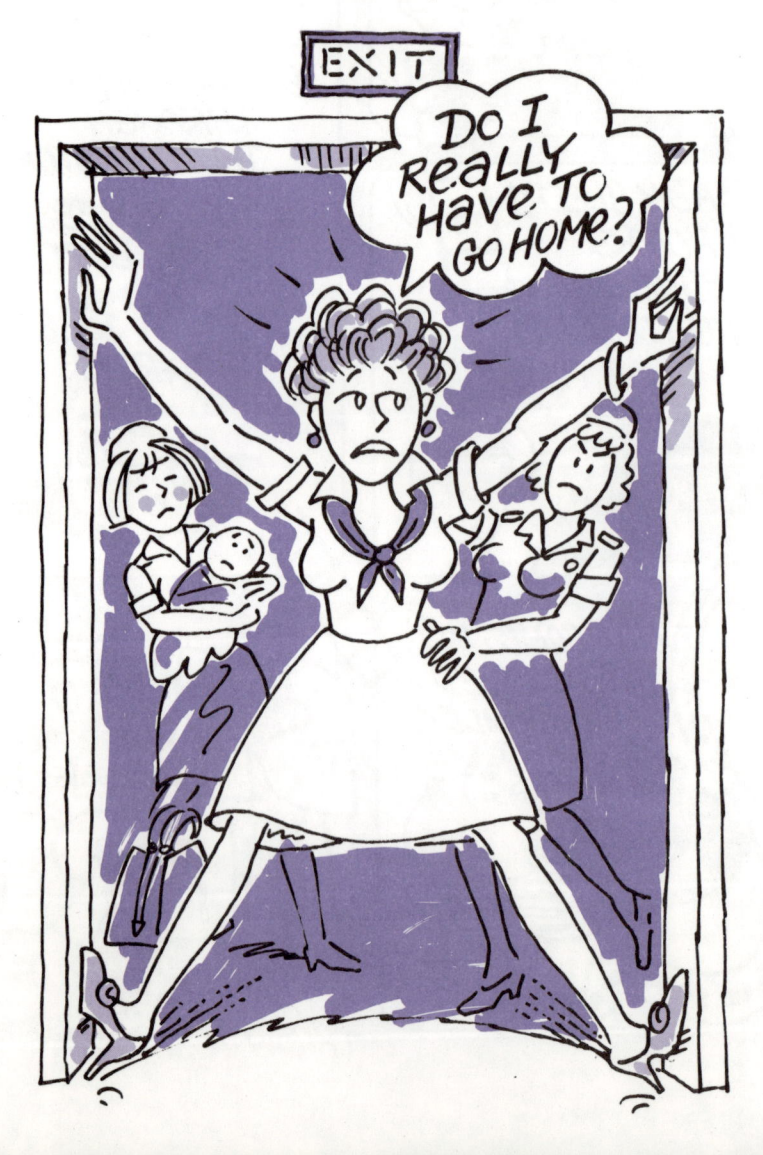

SETTLING IN

personal slave, starts giving this intruder a lot of attention. And to add insult to injury, he regularly sucks on her breasts, which up to now have been your private property.

Your plan of action:
- Become a baby again – demand a dummy and require a day-time nappy.
- Do everything in your power to divert mummy especially during feeds.
- Be as naughty as possible – after all, any attention is better than none.

Bringing home a new baby heralds a major lifestyle change for a hitherto only child and this has to be sympathetically appreciated and planned for by mum and dad.

In the hospital make sure that all the baby's tasks have been done before elder sibling comes at visiting time. This will allow you to spend all of your time and attention on the older child. If the baby cries or plays up, try to ignore the baby or leave it to dad.

When the time comes for you to leave the hospital, big sister or brother should come to help you take the baby home, but should hold *your* hand while dad carries the baby. The worst thing you can do is send the older child away to grandmother when you bring the baby home, in the mistaken belief that it will smooth your return. You will be sending the child a clear message about whom you now prefer.

Use your commonsense and make looking after the baby a joint project. Give the older child a baby doll of their own to look after, and get the child to help with the baby – even if each task takes twice as long. Shower the child with affection. Try to make the older child feel responsible for their little baby. If both are crying at the same time, try to comfort the older sibling first.

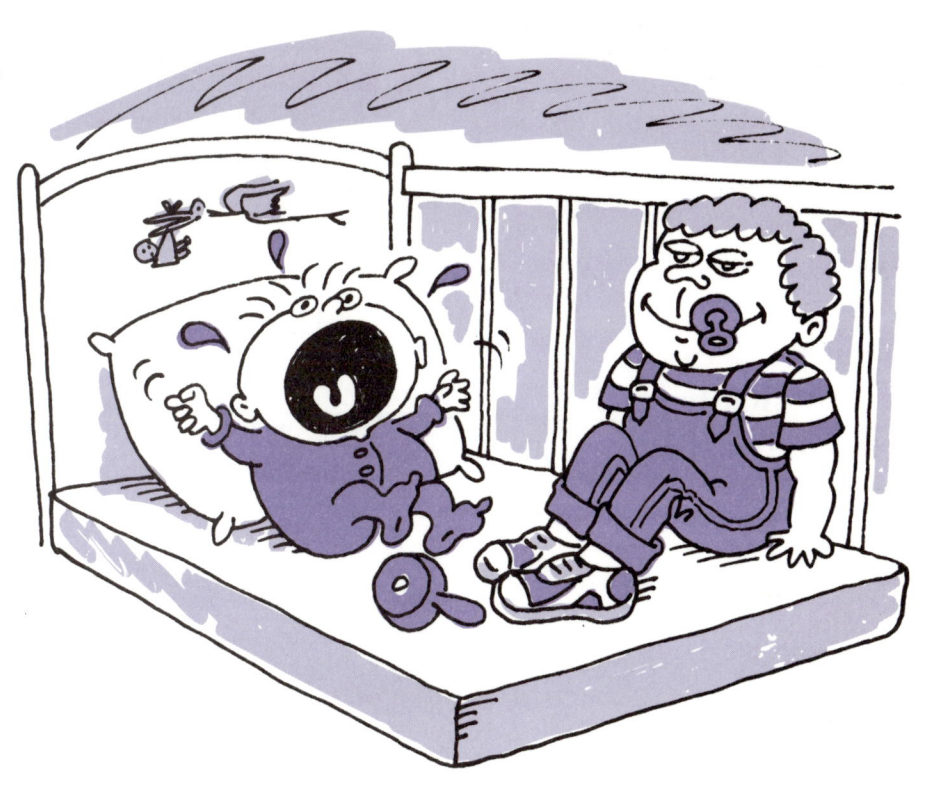

The nearer the child is to three, the easier this will be. Siblings under twenty months do not seem to mind a newcomer as much as the two-year-olds. Two-year-olds are trouble.

FRIENDS

For the first few days after you go home, your real friends will stay away – or if they do show up they bring dinner! As for the others, do not wake the baby for them. Be polite but firm and give them some housework to do. Hopefully they will remember an urgent appointment.

The worst thing you can do is to send the older child to Grandma's when you bring the baby home. This is a clear message about whom you now prefer

55

SETTLING IN

Next to feeding, sleeping is the subject that most concerns new parents (their own as well as their baby's!).

No baby has ever become sick from lack of sleep – only his parents have

SLEEP

The normal baby's requirement of sleep varies enormously but, generally, tired babies sleep. Some babies will sleep twenty-one to twenty-two hours a day and wake only for feeds (these are usually other people's babies!). Other babies may spend most of the daylight hours watching mother, blinking at the light and generally enjoying all the activity around them. Other babies sleep during the day and howl all night. Be reassured that no baby has ever become sick from lack of sleep – only his poor parents have.

Though the family bed has its fans, I would suggest that it is a good idea to have the baby sleeping in his own room right from the early days. Babies are often noisy sleepers, grunting and groaning and many of them also have an interesting breathing rhythm where they pant for a while then stop breathing for up to nine seconds before starting to pant again. This pattern is normal in the first three months of life, but it is a rare parent that can listen to it and get any sleep. By the end of the nine seconds they are usually wide awake and half way to the cot!

Move the cot to the baby's room – you spent all that time decorating it – now use it!

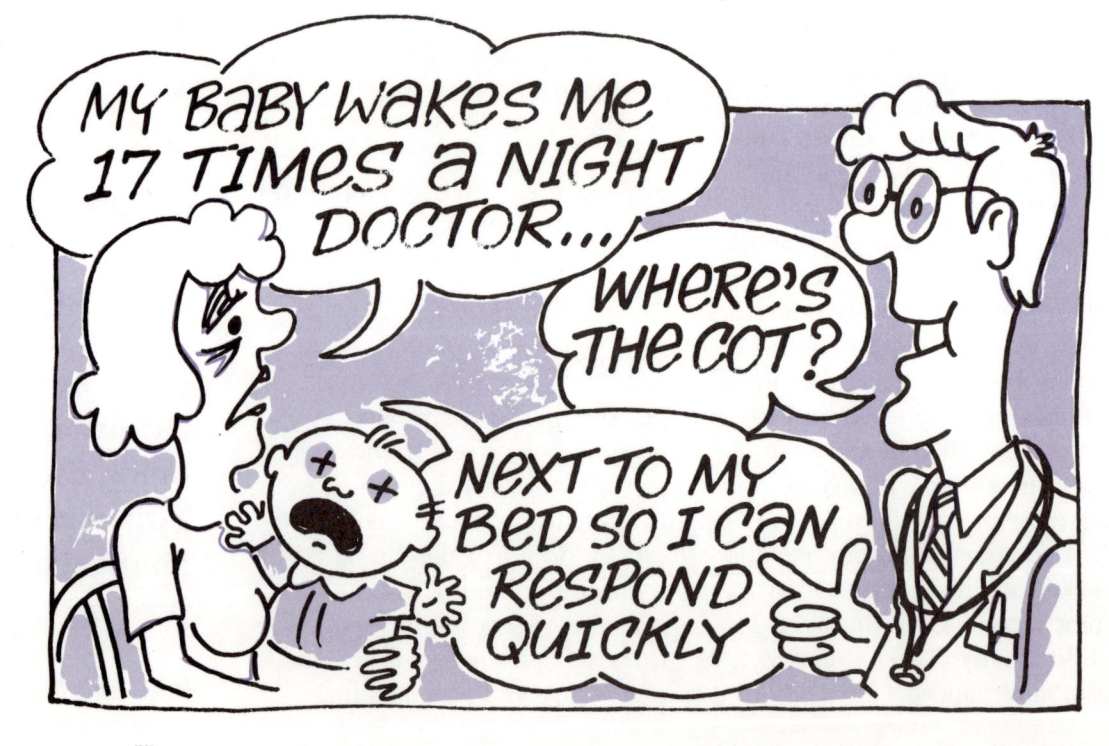

> MY BABY WAKES ME 17 TIMES A NIGHT DOCTOR...
>
> WHERE'S THE COT?
>
> NEXT TO MY BED SO I CAN RESPOND QUICKLY

DEVELOPMENTAL TIMETABLE

At birth your baby lies on his front with his both knees tucked under his abdomen with his head to the side. He tries but cannot lift his head off the mattress. If you turn him over and pull him up by his hands (it's quite safe), his head lags backwards. He has active 'primitive' reflexes. If you tickle the palm of his hand, it will clench in the grasp reflex. If his head is allowed to flop backwards, he will demonstrate a well-developed startle (Moro) reflex in which he throws his arms out. If he is held to stand, he will make clumsy walking movements with his feet, although this is sometimes hard to elicit. He can't yet turn to sound but will gaze fixedly to the light.

At four weeks he intermittently attempts to raise his head from the mattress and on being pulled to sit, has a little head control. His grasp reflex is still present but his other primitive reflexes are starting to disappear. He will now follow your face through a narrow arc and, in the next week or so, he will start to smile back at you if you smile at him first.

At twelve weeks he can look up when lying prone and even push himself up with his hands. When he is pulled to sit, his head is very stable with only an occasional wobble. He starts to notice his hands and will hold on to a rattle which is placed in his hands. He turns his head towards sound and recognises his mother. He has even started to babble conversationally.

At eight weeks he can lift his head off the mattress, when on his front, and his head control is much improved. He has now lost his grasp and walking reflexes and only a part of his startle reflex remains. He can clasp his hands in the midline and can put them in his mouth. His eyes fix and focus and he can follow you with his eyes through a wider arc. He is starting to chuckle and coo.

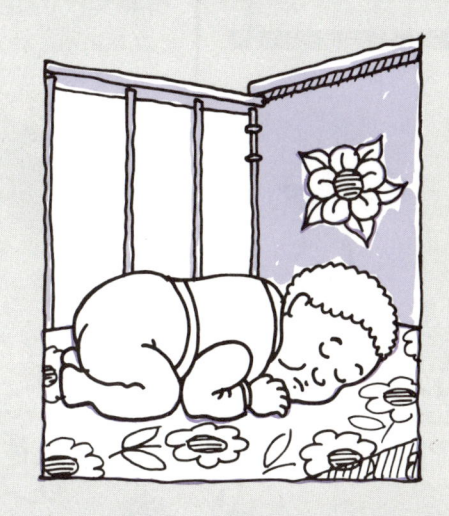

SETTLING IN

The sensitive skin of a newborn baby can be prone to a number of problems, mostly minor ones.

CLOTH VS SINGLE-USE

Studies have shown that single-use nappies do not cause more nappy rash than cloth. If anything they cause fewer problems by more efficiently removing moisture from the skin. However there are two important things to consider before choosing single-use nappies.
1. Putting baby's stools into the garbage rather than the sewage system is not a healthy practice.
2. The plastic covering is not bio-degradable and, unless your area has a high temperature incinerator, it is not possible to dispose of it in an environmentally-friendly way.

NAPPY RASH

Nappy rashes can be divided into three general types:

Contact rash
This rash occurs in those areas in contact with the nappy, leaving the creases of the thighs unaffected. It is mainly caused by irritation of the skin, from moisture in the nappy and also by substances in the urine, like urea, forming ammonia after being broken down by germs from the baby's stool.
Treatment
Wash the nappies in commercial preparations such as Napisan and rinse them carefully, or try disposables for a week or so. Stop using soap on the skin and use a non-soap cleanser with pine tar instead. Use a cream containing zinc and castor oil at first but, if there is no improvement, see your doctor who may prescribe one per cent hydrocortisone cream to use at each nappy change. Once the rash has improved, use a silicone-based barrier cream to protect the skin.

Rash in moist areas
This rash tends to be worse in the creases of the skin, though it may be uniform throughout the nappy area.
Treatment
Use the same management approach as for the contact rash, but in this case the rash may be caused by thrush. See your doctor who may prescribe one per cent hydrocortisone cream and Vioform or some other antifungal antiseptic, such as Daktarin cream.
If either this rash or the contact rash refuses to go away, stop using lanolin altogether, for instance in moist towelettes or baby lotions.

Excoriated buttocks
This rash occurs around the anus and is usually from the stool. The stool of breastfed babies is very acid and, especially if the stool is frothy or fluid, can burn the buttocks.
Treatment
Frequent nappy changing, exposure to the air and one per cent hydrocortisone cream

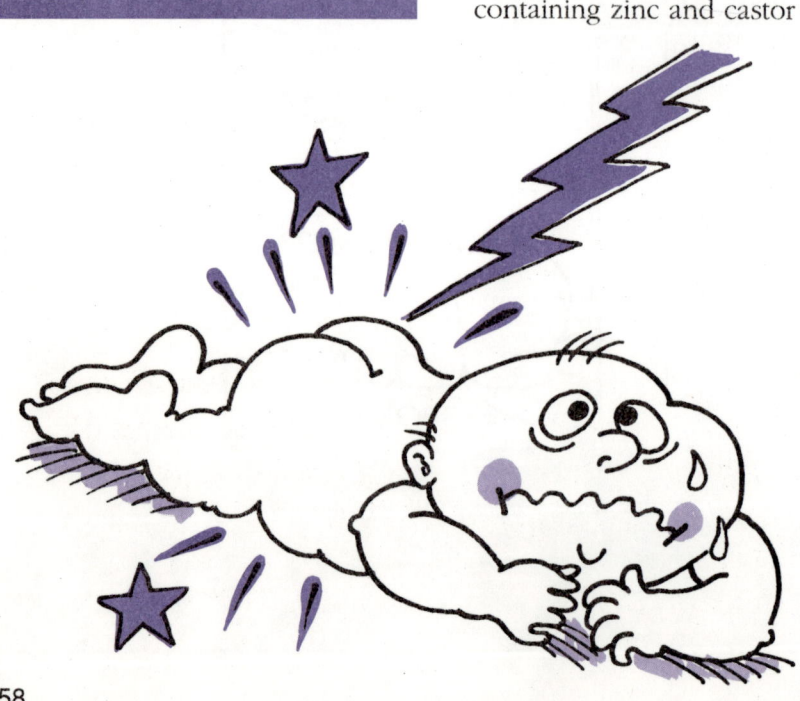

SETTLING IN

should improve matters. A silicone-based barrier cream will protect the skin.

Remember that dermatologists' and paediatricians' babies also get nappy rashes. It does not reflect upon the quality of your care of your baby.

ECZEMA

This characteristic rash occurs in mild form in many babies, usually in the first four months of life. The skin of the cheeks becomes rough and scaly and scaliness of the skin within the hair and eyebrows, called 'cradle-cap', develops. In severe form, the baby can have scaliness, cracking, weeping and redness caused by infection to the skin of most of his upper body, especially behind the ears, back of the neck, face and chest. The conditon is caused by overactivity of the sweat glands and the treatment is directed to diminishing their activity. Babies usually grow out of this tendency in the first six months.

Occasionally in families that are 'atopic', that is, have an allergic tendency, this kind of rash tends to last for longer – even blending into adult-type eczema as the child grows.

To treat the rash, stop using soap for bathing. Instead use a non-soap cleanser containing pine tar. If the rash is severe, limit bathing to a couple of times a week. Avoid the use of fancy baby lotions and creams. Moisturise the skin with sorbolene, with or without glycerin, and use one per cent hydrocortisone in sorbolene cream from your doctor in all but the mildest cases. This steroid cream is very mild and perfectly safe for babies and may be used liberally. It is the mainstay of the treatment. Avoid the use of brushed synthetic fibres or wool next to the skin and if the rash is more than mild, it is best to have it treated by your doctor.

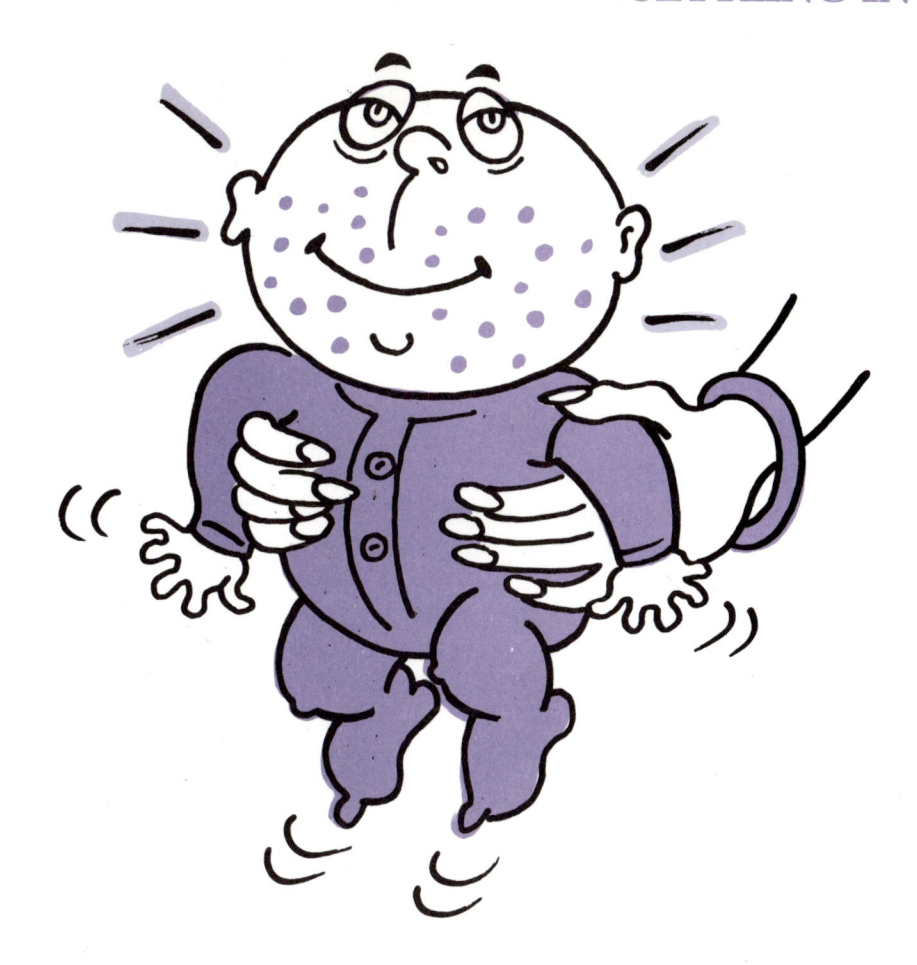

Cradle cap

Cradle cap responds well to petroleum jelly (Vaseline) which softens scales and allows their removal. It is worthwhile trying a tiny amount of anti-dandruff shampoo now and again as this is also likely to help.

SUN KICKS

The days of worshipping the sun are numbered. Sunlight should come with a warning: 'This

'Why is it that as soon as I want to show off my baby, he gets spotty?'

SETTLING IN

All new babies reflux to some degree but most mothers and babies struggle through and the problem disappears

radiation is harmful to your health and, in sufficient dosage, may be lethal'.

Sun kicks are quite helpful to those who live in the northern hemisphere, where the radiation is lower or who have a diet short of vitamin D. It is not relevant somewhere like Australia, where babies should be exposed to the naked rays of the sun as little as possible. When you go out in summer, the baby should always have sunscreen on exposed skin and wear a hat or bonnet with a brim. To see small babies sunbathing naked on beaches is a sad sight – quite apart from the long term aspects of skin cancer, babies can burn badly in minutes. However, it will soon be fashionable to have a porcelain skin (and no wrinkles until you're sixty!).

ORAL THRUSH

Babies have relatively immature immune mechanisms and many of them are not able to withstand infection with a common environmental fungus called Candida albicans, which commonly occurs in the mouth. The infection, better known as thrush, looks like white milk curds stuck to the inside of the cheeks but, unlike milk, they cannot be scraped off. They can also occur on the baby's gums and palate. Thrush can cause soreness but most babies are pretty tolerant of it and it should not cause a feeding problem.

The fungus can be removed effectively by Nystatin or other antifungal medicines (such as Daktarin gel), put in the baby's mouth after he has had a feed. It is also worthwhile putting some antifungal cream (such as Mycostatin) on your nipple if you are breastfeeding to stop cross-infection. If bottle-feeding, be very careful with sterilisation of the bottle and equipment. The thrush is never resistant to these antifungal agents, however it is sometimes difficult to eradicate due to constant re-infection from the feeding equipment. So change the sterilisation fluid you use for dummies, bottles and teats even more often than usual until the infection starts to come under control.

REFLUX

'My baby vomits all the time and brings back EVERYTHING I put into him.'
'Is he putting on weight normally?'
'Yes, but ...'
The mother of a baby who has (gastro-oesophageal) reflux can be recognised by her harassed expression, the nappy permanently on her shoulder and the smell of sour milk that accompanies her wherever she goes.

Frequent vomiting can be a demoralising nuisance. All that beautifully produced milk dumped on the shoulder of your dress or saved for daddy's trousers when he gets home. The vomiting may be effortless or projectile and the baby is often hungry afterwards.

All newborn babies reflux to some degree. There is a valve that lies between the gullet and the stomach which works very poorly in newborns, so the milk may go up and down the gullet like a yo-yo after a feed. In some babies, it comes out of the mouth, in other babies it does

not. The problem with reflux starts when:
- The amount of vomiting becomes more than a nuisance.
- The baby does not put on enough weight.
- People start blaming the baby's crying on the vomiting, saying the baby has 'heartburn' (see 'Colic on page 70).

Reassuringly, the majority of babies will grow out of their reflux problem, usually in the first four months. The question is – can you wait that long?

Initial treatment should be to adjust the baby's resting position. The best posture to empty the stomach and keep the feed as far away from the gullet as possible is with the baby face down and head up at about thirty degrees from the horizontal. For really bad cases, it may be worth propping up the head of the cot on blocks. Some doctors recommend the use of an antacid to decrease the irritation on the lower end of the gullet after each feed. If the reflux is bad in a bottle-fed baby, it is worthwhile thickening up the feeds with carobel or some other thickener. Later on, the introduction of solids can do the same thing. Your doctor can also prescribe some drugs, such as Maxolon or Bethanecol, which help close the valve between the gullet and the stomach, although this probably should not be first-line treatment

Only in the worst cases is an operation to make the valve more efficient necessary and this is extremely rare. Most babies (and their mothers) struggle through this period and the problem disappears.

BOWEL ACTIONS

Breastfed baby
For a breastfed baby it is equally normal, once meconium has been passed and the milk is in, for the baby to have twenty stools a day or one every two weeks. Anything between these two extremes is normal. The

It is as normal for a breastfed baby to have twenty stools a day as one every two weeks. Anything between these two extremes is normal

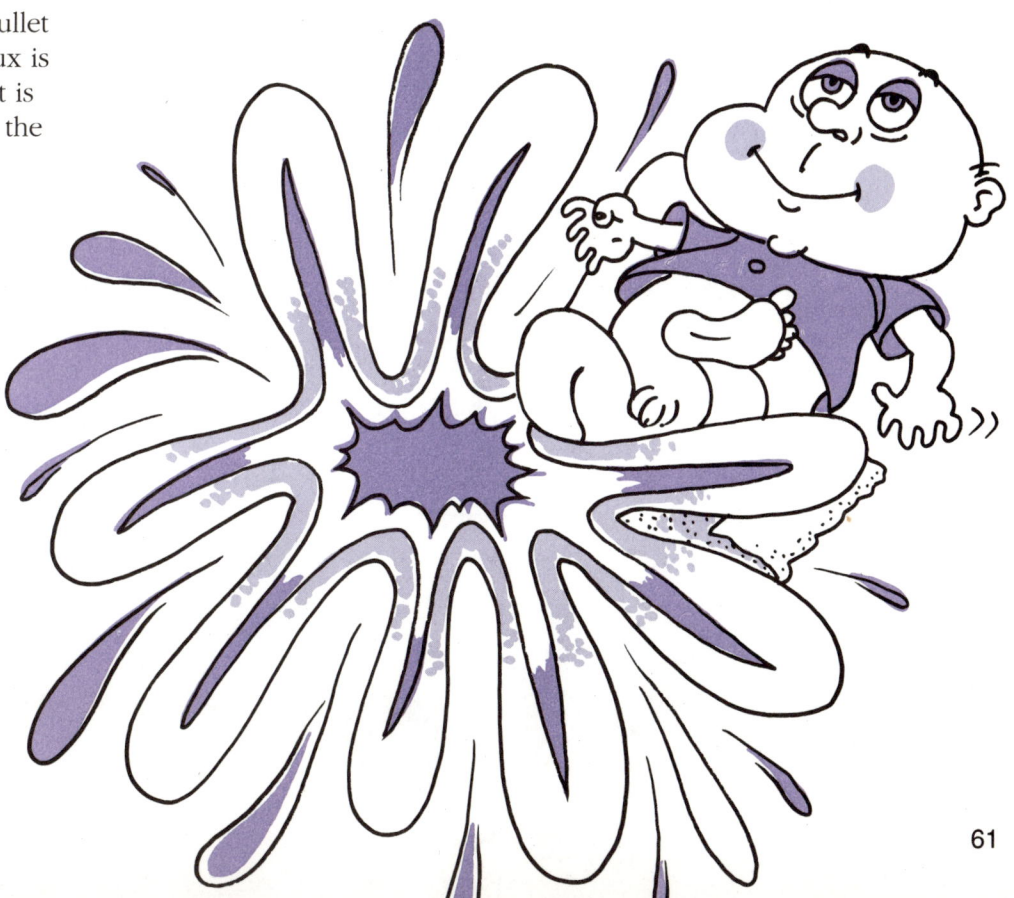

SETTLING IN

Breastfed babies have immunity to bacterial gastroenteritis but viral disease can still occur

stool can be yellow, green, brown, or any combination of these. It can be frankly fluid, seedy or pasty. For breastfed babies, it is never hard. I have never met a normal breastfed baby who is constipated, that is, passing hard stools. If you are worried that your baby has not passed a stool for several days, when he eventually does pass it, you can be reassured by its consistency. If he is passing anything other than rabbit pellets it is normal.

Breastfed babies can seem uncomfortable on the day, or perhaps the day before, they produce less frequent stools. You will soon get to know your baby's particular patterns and accept this as quite normal. Breastfed babies NEVER need any help to go more frequently.

The only stool that should cause you concern is when it is so watery it resembles urine. Under these circumstances it is wise to seek medical advice as the baby may have gastroenteritis. Breastfed babies have immunity to bacterial gastroenteritis, but viral disease can still occur.

The baby producing the loose frequent stools is often the baby who is spilling a little sugar of milk (lactose) in the stool. This is a normal finding and does not represent 'lactose intolerance'.

Bottle-fed baby
Bottle-fed babies tend to have rather firmer stools and to pass them between four times a day and once every two days. The colour tends more to the rustic browns and greens rather than the Van Gogh yellow. It is certainly possible for them to become constipated but again the diagnosis rests on the fact of hard stools rather than infrequency. If the stool is firm or hard, adding a little maltogen or brown sugar (one to two teaspoons to a bottle) or offering a small amount of prune juice will normally be sufficient to soften it. Sometimes well-diluted orange juice and extra water will be helpful. Don't be tempted to use suppositories for your baby unless you check with your doctor – it is almost never necessary.

Loose, watery stools in the bottle-fed baby should be treated with respect as there is a risk of gastroenteritis. So go and see your doctor and take a sample of the stool with you. To collect one, line a nappy with a plastic bag so the fluid is also caught. If you have to wait very long for the stool, it's probably all right anyway!

OUT AND ABOUT

Driving
It is incredible the number of unrestrained children one can see in the back, or worse, in the front seats of cars. These pre-

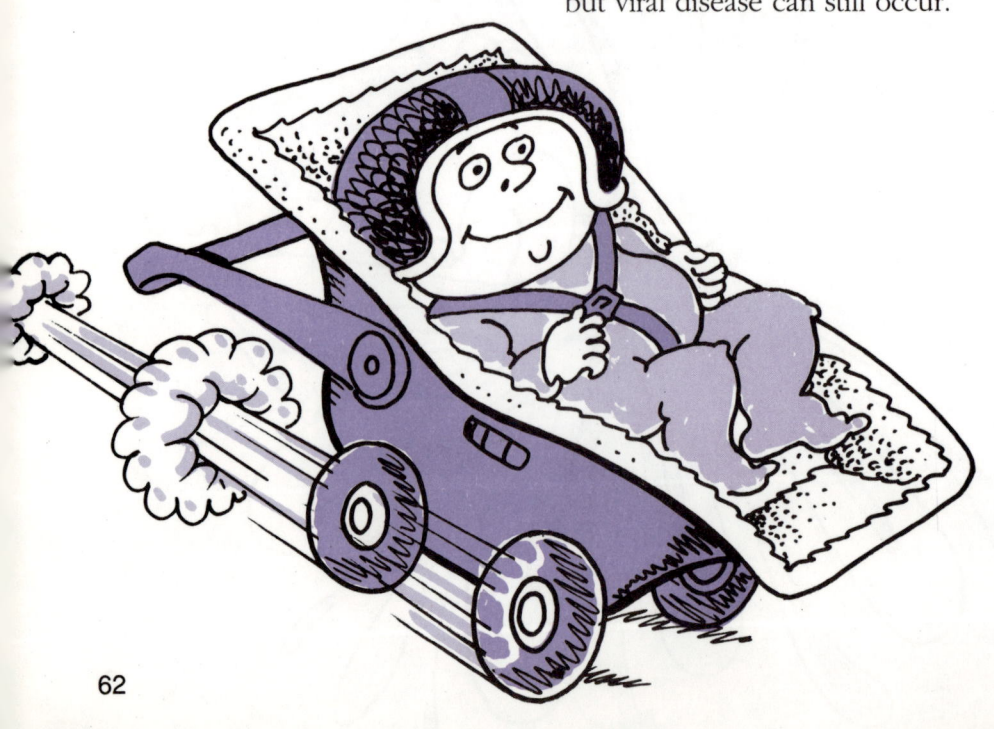

SETTLING IN

sumably loving parents are obviously unaware that with the slightest deceleration of the car their child becomes a missile so heavy that the strongest man could not hold on to him. Anyone who has worked in a children's intensive care unit for a short time will tell you of the agony of parents who are completely unharmed after a minor collision and whose child has gone through the windscreen and now lies broken or dying in hospital. No journey is so short that a child should be unrestrained. Remember most road accidents occur within a short distance of home.

It is now mandatory by law that your baby must always travel in a restraint device in a car. The best one is a rear-facing safety capsule. Get it fitted as soon as, or before, you go into labour so that it is all ready to take your baby home from hospital. Quite apart from the safety aspect of the first drive home, it gets you into the habit of never having children or babies in the car unless they are fully restrained.

As your child grows, if he strongly resents being strapped in, then it is a very good time to teach him some discipline and for him to realise that some rules are unchanging and not open to negotiation.

Like child abuse, there is never any excuse.

Flying

Airliners are pressurised to an atmospheric pressure equal to that at five thousand feet so that it is perfectly safe to take even your newborn baby to see his relatives overseas. Beware only if he was born prematurely and had severe lung disease.

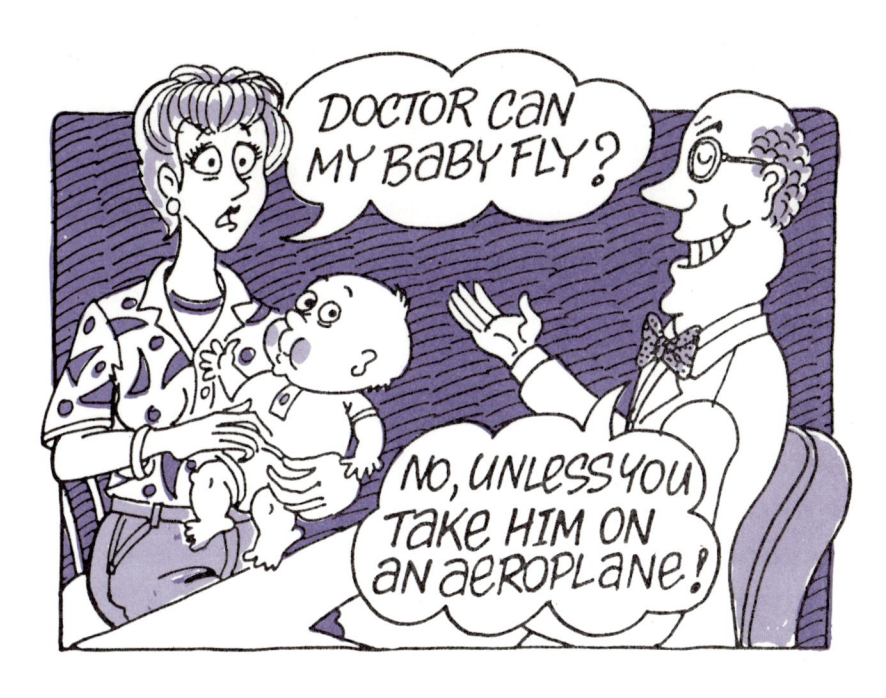

It is, in fact, a good deal easier to travel with a newborn baby than it is with a toddler. Babies do not have the constant need to move around and can usually be comforted with the breast or a feed. They also do not kick the chair in front, spill every drink handed to them, need to go to the toilet only when the food trolleys are blocking all the aisles or become fascinated with the hair of the man in the seat in front.

Pressure problems in the middle ear on descending are probably less common in babies than they are in adults, as the eustachian (connecting) tube between the pharynx and the middle ear is much shorter. Nevertheless, when the plane descends, it is worthwhile getting the baby to suck as this will equalise pressures around the eardrum. Unfortunately, pilots do not always tell you when they start their descent, which is often an hour before arrival, so be ready.

Strictly speaking, it does not really matter if the baby becomes upset because of the pressure in his ears because he will yell and that is precisely the best treatment to equalise the pressure. His noise should not worry your fellow passengers as their ears will also be affected by the descent!

No journey is so short that a child should be unrestrained. Most road accidents occur close to home

63

SETTLING IN

Except for a few special circumstances, every child should be fully immunised. Anything you may have heard to the contrary is unbalanced and untrue.

Whooping cough is a far more common cause of death or permanent damage than immunisation

IMMUNISATION

The only contraindications to immunisation are:
- If your baby has a congenital immune deficient disease.
- If your baby suffers a serious neurological disorder or has a history of convulsions or both.
- If your baby has suffered a reaction to vaccine (usually the pertussis vaccine) so serious that it required hospitalisation, such as a temperature of more than 40°C (104°F), a fit or a major shock or allergic reaction.

Most babies will develop a slight fever and be somewhat irritable for a day or two following the triple antigen vaccination. In addition, there may be some local reaction, such as redness at the site of injection. Such reactions are not a contra-indication to further dosage.

Although it is not a good idea to immunise your baby if he is in the throes of a viral infection, this does not include minor infections of the upper respiratory tract. It is perfectly fine to vaccinate your baby if he has a runny nose and a cough. Some babies have snuffles which last for months and immunisation shouldn't be delayed without a good excuse.

The dangers of immunisation have been largely overstated. The only vaccine with important side effects is that of whooping cough (pertussis). One in over three hundred thousand babies who are immunised with this vaccine will develop a damaging neurological disease which is permanent. However, two important points are made by the National Childhood Encephalopathy Study from the UK, a nationwide study on the risks of pertussis vaccination:

1 The risk to babies is likely to be even lower than the figure given above – especially if contraindications are adhered to.
2 Whooping cough is a far more common cause of death or permanent neurological damage in babies than the immunisation. There is usually an outbreak of whooping cough in Australia or

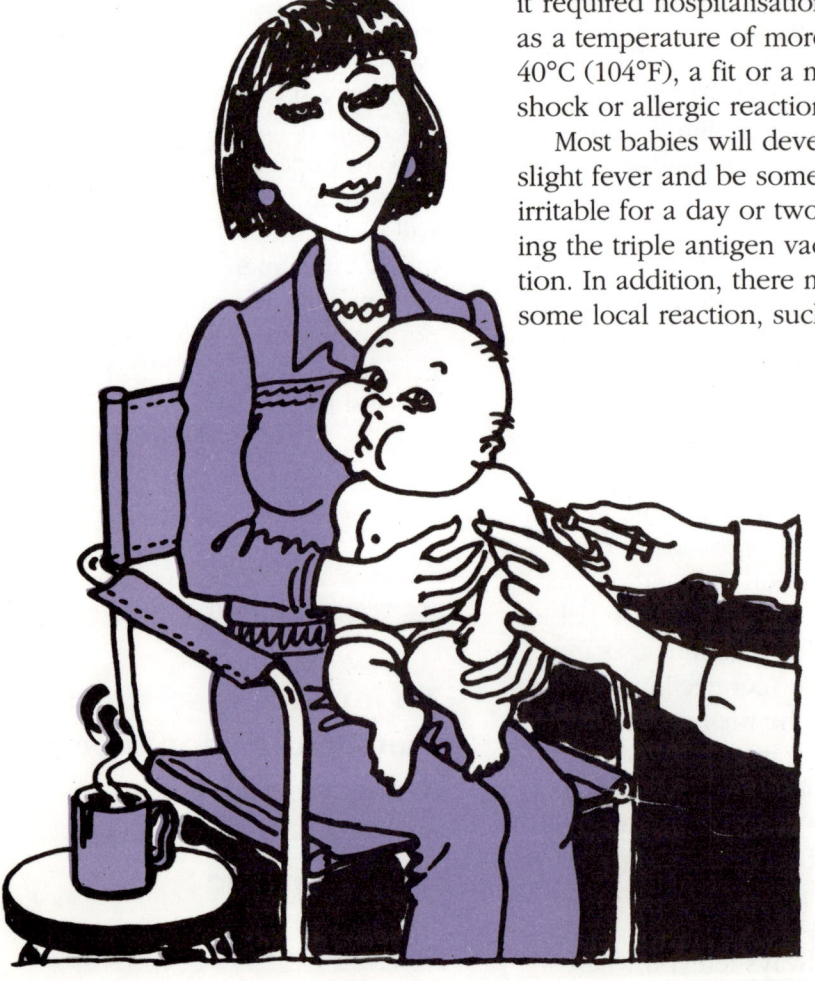

SETTLING IN

the UK every few years just to remind us all how serious the disease can be. During these outbreaks the death rate from whooping cough can be as high as one in five hundred cases for babies under one year.

After your baby receives his 'triple' injections, it is worthwhile giving him a dose of paracetamol elixir four-hourly as a routine for the first twelve hours if he is awake. This is all that should be required.

Last but not least, there is absolutely no scientific evidence that so-called 'homoeopathic immunisation' bestows anything except a false sense of security.

Hepatitis B immunisation

The latest Hepatitis B vaccines are synthetic and completely safe. Hepatitis B is a potentially fatal viral infection of the liver which can be obtained from stepping on needles used by infected drug addicts or from close contact with carriers of the virus. The introduction of this vaccine is a real breakthrough in medical technology and a godsend to us all. It is worthwhile considering giving to yourself, your baby and your whole family, even if you do not consider yourself in a high-risk category. It is perfectly safe for babies and the program is for three injections, the first at birth, the second one month later and the third six months after the first. There is rarely any reaction.

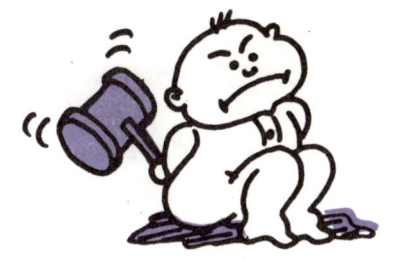

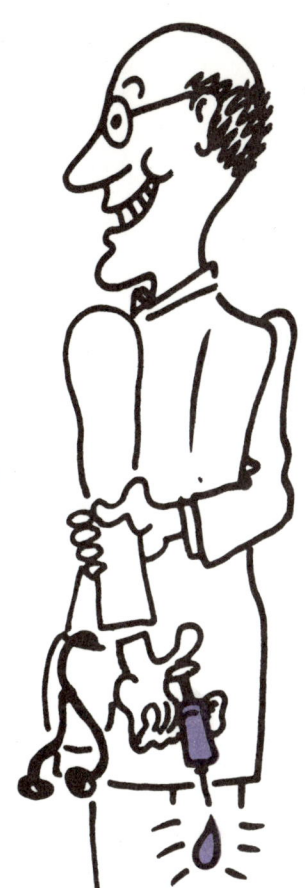

IMMUNISATION TIMETABLE

Specific times for vaccination of new babies varies a little according to where you live but the following table is a useful guide.

2 months	triple antigen: diphtheria, pertussis (whooping cough) and tetanus (DPT)
4 months	triple antigen (DPT), Sabin (polio)
6 months	triple antigen (DPT), Sabin (polio)
15 months	measles, mumps
18 months	triple antigen (DPT)
Pre-school	double antigen: diphtheria, tetanus (CDT), Sabin (polio)

SETTLING IN

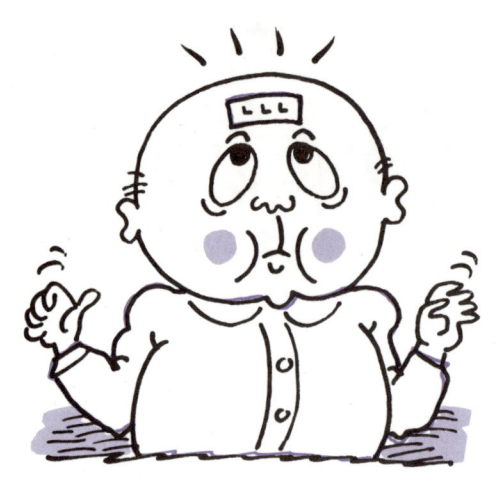

FEVERS, COUGHS AND COLDS

'The entire family has the flu and now the baby's developed snuffles.'

Newborn babies who are breastfed rarely get infections of the upper respiratory tract (coughs and colds). There are antiviral substances in the breastmilk that have a protective effect. Indeed, in the case of middle ear infection, the effect seems to last even after the baby has been weaned and the breastfeeding only lasted a few weeks. That is NOT to say that the baby will not develop snuffles (see section on 'Snuffles' on page 32).

Having said that, it is still possible for your baby to catch a cold, especially if the baby's older brother or sister is going to playgroup or preschool and bringing home all the viruses that are going around. If your baby has snuffles and a temperature then it is probably due to a viral infection. The normal underarm temperature for your baby is 36.5°C (97.8°F). Any temperature over 37°C (98.6°F) is probably significant. However, the management of a cold, flu or a mild cough is purely to treat just the symptoms. There are no antibiotics or drugs that can kill viruses. We must wait until the baby's immune mechanism fixes the problem by itself.

However, to control a high temperature, a baby paracetamol elixir is very useful and may be given in the correct dosage for the baby's age, every four hours. However, this dosage must not be exceeded. If the baby has a blocked nose bad enough to interfere with feeding, a drop of nasal antihistamine decongestant can clear it for long enough to get a feed down. Nasal decongestants should not be used regularly, however, except under medical advice. Anyway, it is a good idea to have your doctor check to make sure that there is no middle ear or chest infection.

Temperatures over 38° C (100.4°F) should be treated with respect and the baby taken to the doctor for diagnosis. If in the presence of a diagnosed viral illness, the temperature continues to stay high, the baby should be treated with paracetamol elixir regularly, or if this is not enough, sponging with lukewarm water helps to bring the temperature down. Do not use cold water as it is less effective for extracting warmth from the baby's body. To take the baby's temperature, use a mercury thermometer under his armpit or the stick-on ones for his forehead.

Respiratory viral infections normally right themselves in a few days but if your baby develops a wheeze, a seal-like bark or a 'smokers cough' see your doctor straight away.

To take the baby's temperature, use a mercury thermometer under his armpit, or a stick-on one for his forehead

SETTLING IN

WHEN TO CALL THE DOCTOR

Babies have countless ways of worrying their parents and it is important at these times to remember that there is a great range of normal behaviour. All new parents are naturally anxious about their baby's health, and it is easy to overreact. On most occasions, no intervention is necessary. However, if your baby exhibits **any** of the following signs or symptoms get your doctor to check things out.

- Baby's respiratory rate is sixty or more per minute maintained over five minutes or more

- Temperatures greater than 39°C (102.2°F) or below 36°C (96.8°F)

- Fits or convulsions

- Fewer than two wet nappies per day

- Increasing jaundice beyond one week of age

- Blood in stool or urine beyond one week of age

- Pale, listless baby

- Baby refuses all feeds

- Combination of vomiting and watery diarrhoea

- Repeated projectile vomiting

- Symmetrical red inflammation around the base of the stump of the umbilical cord

- The baby has difficulty breathing

- Barking seal-like cough

- Baby does not move limbs symmetrically

- Baby doesn't look right

SETTLING IN

Every parent whose baby first sleeps through the night experiences a hollow feeling as they go to check that their baby is breathing

COT DEATH

Nothing strikes fear into the hearts of new parents quite like cot death. The problem is that we are virtually helpless to prevent it. Luckily, however, it is really quite rare. About two in a thousand babies are lost in this unexpected and insidious way. By definition, the babies die quietly, without a struggle, during sleep.

Statistics tell us that it more commonly occurs in boys than girls, during cold months rather than warm months of the year, to babies mostly under eighteen months (maximally at about two months of age), and to bottle-fed babies who may have an upper respiratory tract infection at the time. There may be (although this has been recently disputed) an increased incidence in the siblings of those who have died in this way. The incidence seems to be slightly increased in babies who are born prematurely or those of narcotic-addicted mothers.

You can paper the walls with theories as to the cause but basically it probably comes down to a failure of the breathing drive. Feeding into this final common pathway are many factors, some genetic, some not, and nobody has yet come near to satisfactorily unravelling the web of combining factors to explain all cases. Nevertheless two of these are worth noting, even at our present level of knowledge.

• The front-down or prone posture of an infant in the cot seems to be less safe than that on the side or even the back.
• The factor of high temperature caused by a fever with too warm an environment or over-wrapping may contribute.

Though clearly these are not anything like complete explanations they are probably worth noting until more information is available.

Monitoring

No-one has shown satisfactorily that the electronic monitoring of babies makes any difference. Some babies fire off the alarm because they stop breathing, but no-one knows whether they would have gone on to die if left alone, or whether this 'apnoea' (Latin for 'no breathing') attack is even the same condition. Also, babies still die of cot death while being monitored – by the time the monitor alarm goes off many of them cannot be revived.

We all share the same fear – paediatrician and printer, bus driver and journalist. Every parent whose baby first sleeps through the night will remember the hollow feeling in the stomach as they walk towards the baby's room to check that their baby is still breathing. As already mentioned, it is not worthwhile electronically monitoring babies who have no special risks. There are usually too many terrifying false alarms and the monitor is no guarantee of preventing cot death. For very anxious parents a monitor may decrease the anxiety and for those it is an option to discuss with the paediatrician. I have seen some parents who would otherwise have watched the baby in shifts and never slept together again until the baby was two, but such anxiety is very rare.

My suggestions are therefore:

SETTLING IN

- Think about it as little as possible.
- Buy an intercom (a simple wire one is not expensive, a radiotransmitter type will cost a lot more).
- Get your baby used to sleeping on his side.
- Avoid overwrapping your baby with blankets or warming his room too much, especially if he has a cold or other infection. An ideal room temperature is about 18°C (64°F).

It is likely that in the future we will discover that there is an inborn propensity for some infants to stop breathing in this way and the external factors just trigger the event. Research is now under way in many countries to find such an inborn error and hence a screening test. Until that day comes, just keep on remembering that the danger of cot death is less than that of crossing the road.

MOTHER NOT MARTYR

Throughout the whole wonderful experience of getting to know your baby in the first few weeks, it is critically important that you do not forget two very important people – yourself and your partner. It takes some effort to juggle everyone's needs and take care of yourself at the same time in this situation. Eat normally and regularly. If you are breastfeeding, your weight should diminish anyway as you transfer your fat deposits to the baby and it is important to have a good nourishing diet to provide for you both.

If you are obsessive about housework then try to get some help. This is no time to clean, wash and scrub. If you can't arrange some help, let the house go just a little and enjoy the little spare time you have.

As fathers have not gone through delivery, they may not fully understand that it takes some weeks for you to recover your strength, quite apart from the nocturnal demands made on you by a little baby. Sex may be the last thing on your mind in these first weeks, but do not forget that it may be uppermost in your husband's. The most vital sexual activity for you both at this time is to talk about it and not just avoid the subject. Then when your libido starts to return you don't find a cranky, jealous mate who feels he's been jilted in favour of a baby.

Babies have a few critical needs and the most important is a happy mother and father in a stable loving relationship. This aspect of baby care needs as much attention as the nappies.

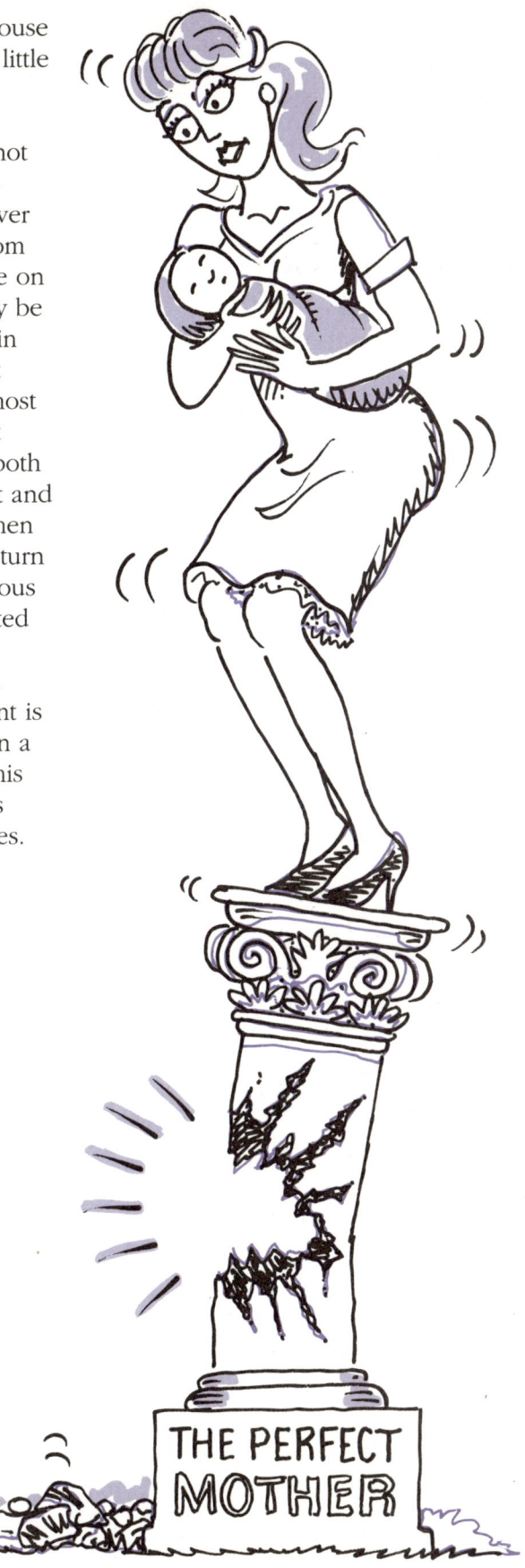

THE PERFECT MOTHER

COLIC AND THE CRYING BABY

Whenever a baby cries for no apparent reason and won't stop, it is likely to be labelled 'colic' or 'wind'. Even more so if his legs are drawn up to his tummy as he yells, if he passes a lot of wind or, if picked up, can be burped.

Most old beliefs about colic and crying are just myths and acting on them often makes matters worse

If the bouts of crying start occurring frequently parents usually notice that a pattern emerges and start searching frantically for a cause. Then comes the avalanche of advice. It is incredible to hear the advice given to these poor unfortunate parents.

Everything from 'tummy massages', 'a drop of brandy' to the saddest suggestion of all, 'put him on the bottle'.

All useless, all untrue but frantic, tired parents are an easy target for these 'helpful people'.

At its most severe, descriptions of events from different parents are remarkably similar, so there is no doubt that 'colic' exists. It tends to recur at certain times of the day, most commonly in the evening – hence 'six o'clock colic'. During the attacks the baby appears uncomfortable and squirms, drawing his knees up and crying or even screaming, with apparent pain. Occasionally he will waken out of a deep sleep with a 'jump' and this will precede a bout of crying. The smallest thing can trigger off the attacks – passing wind, wetting his nappy, or just 'being bored'. Sometimes they occur around feed times, with the baby pulling off the breast and screaming.

The attacks may be relieved by picking him up, cuddling and feeding, or vigorous sucking on a dummy. Occasionally the baby will calm down when he is driven around in a car but often nothing helps at all.

Not surprisingly, the situation can create enormous domestic tension. There is something about the incessant crying of a baby that drives even the most even-tempered people up the wall. Soon both parents are at the end of their tether, sleepless, frustrated, angry and guilty. Guilty about the anger they feel at this ungrateful little being, for whom so much is done for so little reward.

At the outset it is important to realise that most old beliefs about colic and crying are just myths and acting on them often makes matters worse.

Firstly, babies who cry will swallow air. The wind does not cause the crying – the crying causes the wind.

Secondly, 'colicky' babies and their parents are perfectly normal people, with no special allergies or psychological problems – except those caused by a baby screaming at them for a few weeks!

Thirdly, in nearly all cases there is nothing whatever the matter with the baby's tummy. Any baby who gives a vigorous cry is liable to draw his knees up – this gives a bit more power

COLIC AND THE CRYING BABY

to the yell, it is not that he's got a pain. When one thinks about it, it is quite illogical that a breastfed baby, fed with the most physiologically pure food available, should develop a tummy ache from it. Nature is usually a bit more efficient than that! Also, parents often notice that the crying is worse at a particular time of the day – often the evening. As babies are fed on a twenty-four hour clock it is unlikely to be the fault of the feed or his tummy.

There is a newer scapegoat. Reflux heartburn is often now given the blame and treatment with antacids recommended. However radiologically proven refluxing babies mostly do not suffer 'colic'.

If the baby has a bit of lactose intolerance (see page 50) and has loose stools and a gurgly tummy, then usually this is blamed for the 'pain'. However there is an equal number of comfortable babies with similar stools and research studies are far from convincing.

So the breastfed baby does not need the bottle and the bottle-fed baby does not need his formula changed. Neither does he have distension or spasm in his gut. All these particular myths have been perpetuated through history because of the baby's appearance and behaviour, and you can't blame anyone for being fooled.

It is fairly certain now that in most cases the basic cause of the whole problem is tension, anxiety, or stress in the baby.

Why should a baby be tense?
When the baby is in the womb he gently floats around in a sea of warm soothing water in perfect peace. Following delivery, things are very different. His life is now more noisy and active. He has hunger, thirst, discomfort and fatigue. His posture is no longer contained, secure and snug. He is no longer a physical part of his mother. Depending on the baby's personality he may find all of this very hard to tolerate and react accordingly.

On top of the actual abrupt life changes there is an additional compelling factor that causes babies to be subject to stress. Research with premature babies has shown that they, and to a lesser extent term babies, are very susceptible to overstimulation. Things such as noise, activity, disruption or stress in the home atmosphere may arouse and stimulate a baby. However the most powerful stimulus is human contact, and especially, eye contact.

Think about how we usually approach a baby. Most people gaze deep into his eyes, and make noises to attract his attention and get him to gaze back. Unfortunately a lot of such intense eye contact can be very stressful for a young baby. It really excites him. It would be all right if he could just switch off the input, as older people do, when he has had enough. Alas, babies just can't do this. They are excited and 'stressed' and they cry. This is one clear explanation why this problem occurs more in the evenings.

When a baby cries it is normal and appropriate for his parents to become anxious and concerned about him. We know from research that a baby's cry is imprinted into his mother's mind within a few hours of birth. His

Intense eye contact can be very stressful for a young baby

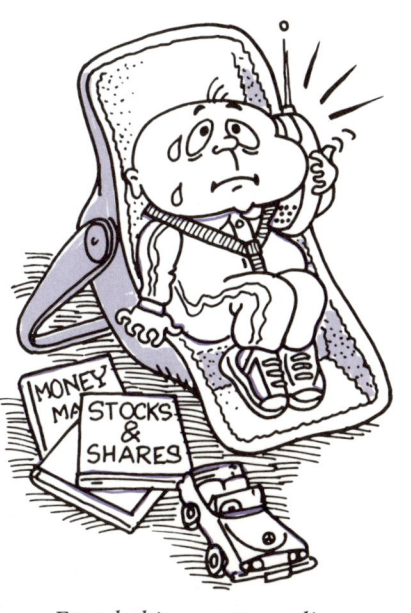

Even babies get stressed!

COLIC AND THE CRYING BABY

cry then acts as an 'arousal mechanism' over which she has little control. It is not only normal for a mother to become agitated and to wake out of the deepest sleep when her baby cries, it is a fundamental survival reflex for the baby. This maternal instinct sends the mother into a frenzy of activity, finding out what is wrong and meeting the baby's needs to stop him crying. But as babies are very sensitive to stress from their surroundings, this very activity can make them more anxious and make them cry even more. This makes mother more anxious, more active and makes **her** cry more! Round and round this vicious circle goes, driving both into intense anguish and misery.

Even more directly, the parents' response is often to go to the baby, pick him up, look him in the eyes and ask him what the problem is. This is like putting the rock music back on and the baby just keeps on dancing! What he is really saying is 'PLEASE LEAVE ME ALONE!' and that is precisely what they are not doing.

Clearly some babies are better at handling such stimulation than others. The variable is the baby's personality. Some can cope, and others can't, at least for a few months until they learn to switch off. Most babies will grow out of this problem by about four months of age. So hang in there!

What do we do about it?

In the early stages it is often enough for mum and dad to realise what is going on to control the problem. If you realise that, if anything, there is too much parenting rather than too little in your family and the baby's cries don't represent intense agony, pain or a rejection of your love then you are more able to think straight about the problem.

First, listen to your baby's different cries. I'm sure there are several. A hungry one (loud and insistent), a tired one (mumble, mumble, bleat), need a cuddle, (waa, waa, waa), and so on right through to the mind-wrenching scream of the over-stressed, anxious or insecure baby. Try to sort them out and 'tune in' to what's behind them. Stop a while and think before reacting. Get to know your baby's other signals. Hiccupping is commonly a sign of a full stomach but sometimes is a sign of agitation and stress. Yawning, straining and pushing with the limbs are signs that the baby may be overloaded with stimuli and would prefer a period of peace and quiet.

If there's any possibility that the cry may be a hungry one, feed him. If you're wrong, he may not be interested or may vomit, it doesn't matter either way. You'll know next time and it's important to eliminate this cause of crying before we move onto other things. Overfeeding is not a problem in the short term, so don't worry about it.

Once that possibility is out of the way, we can turn to more subtle things. Try to make your infant feel as snug and secure as possible. Swaddling is a good technique. It works even better if the wrapping persuades the baby to lie like a fetus, with the back rounded and head forward slightly, shoulders hunched, arms and legs flexed towards the body. This gives the baby a

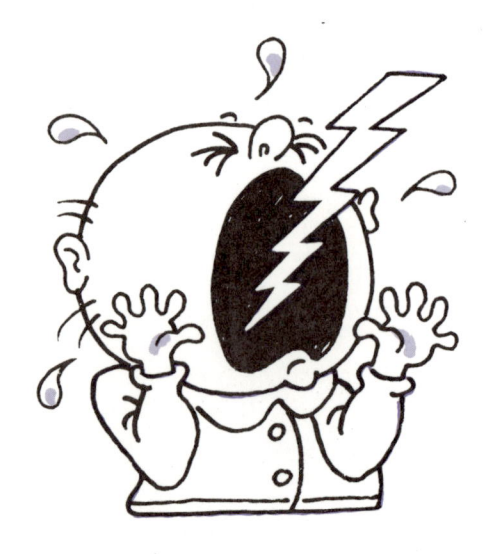

Learn to recognise your baby's various cries and respond accordingly

COLIC AND THE CRYING BABY

sense of security. The swaddling should be firm enough so the hands, shoulders and legs are all contained. Lying the baby on his side whilst swaddled will also help to encourage sleep.

Hold him until he relaxes. Often these stressed babies resist the swaddling and fight to get their arms and legs free so they can flail them around. This is very upsetting for them and should be resisted. Gentle but firm persuasion should keep the limbs contained in the blanket. To calm him use dim lights and a gentle voice. Avoid too much eye-contact and don't overload him with your voice, rocking and looking at him all at once.

Once he settles, place him on his side or front in his cot and, at an early opportunity, vacate the area. If he starts crying, again, don't go in straight away but see if he calms down by himself. If he does not, repeat the swaddling and calming, soften his environment as much as possible by relaxed, slow movements and again leave as soon as he settles.

It is critical to understand that it is all right to leave the baby once he has settled a little. If he has been fed, changed and cuddled and still he continues to cry, then it is best for him that you don't get 'sucked in' any further. From here on you should do whatever calms YOU the most. If that is to carry him around – that's all right. But equally, if it is to leave him in his cot to cry and get yourself a stiff drink, then that's all right too. Remember crying is a great de-stressor – it may be just what your baby needs to calm down.

There comes a time when you know that your presence is not helping. Indeed, you may find that when you pick him up he will stiffen and his cries will increase. He is saying 'Please leave me alone, I've had enough for one day!' Don't hover outside the door, wringing your hands, as he can sense you out there. Try to get out of earshot for a while, before going back to check on him.

How long you leave him depends on two things – him and you! If he starts really screaming again, go in and calm him before settling him again on his own. If you find it difficult not to go in when your baby cries, leave him for ten minutes or so before going in to check on him. When you do go in, don't turn on the light, and avoid eye-contact with him.

There are other techniques worth a try.

- Relaxation baths will often calm an excited baby down. The water is ideally about twenty centimetres deep and the usual warm temperature. Instead of bathing the baby on his back and supporting the back of his head, which allows his arms to fling out as he startles, float him on his front with a hand under his chin to keep his head out of the water. The water must be deep enough so he does not touch the bottom, but floats gently on the surface. Many babies promptly go to sleep when immersed in this way.
- Carrying babies around in a pouch often provides a comforting environment for the brittle-tempered baby, allowing him to be held against his mother's chest while leaving her arms free. Babies usually calm rapidly when carried this way.
- If the baby finds comfort in sucking, let him. Whatever your prejudices about dummies, this is one situation when they should be buried.
- For dog-tired parents, help from a third party can give them the sleep they so badly need to get their confidence back and allow a more balanced view of the situation. So ask grandmother over for the weekend- she may enjoy being needed, despite the noise!
- Sometimes a small dose of sedative for the baby will help to calm him. (When anti-colic medicines work it is because they are sedatives).
- Moving mother and baby to a residential mothercraft home, if one is available, almost always solves the problem.

The lesson of self-calming (clinical psychologists call the process 'returning to base') is an important one for a baby to learn in the first few months of life. When he is calm, he can then get on with the next task, that of learning to concentrate.

The only other important fact to remember is that no young baby has ever damaged himself from crying, either physically or emotionally. Whatever else they are, babies are superbly designed crying machines who can, and occasionally do, cry for hours non-stop without harming anyone but their parents!

LOSING A LITTLE, LOSING IT ALL

To a greater or lesser extent, being delivered of a baby with a congenital malformation or, even worse, suffering the loss of a baby, sets in train the grieving process. Its function is to help us adjust and recover and go back to living our lives in fullness and contentment.

Giving birth to a less than perfect baby is a deeply disappointing event and one that all prospective parents secretly fear

The first response to this kind of tragedy is often total disbelief. Our mind plays tricks on us, telling us that it is not true and that we will soon wake up and all will be well. Alas, soon this numbness wears off to be replaced by anger and sadness. We feel cheated that this could have happened to our baby. We examine the pregnancy in minute detail to try and find a reason, and even though there often is none, the feeling of responsibility and guilt remains.

CONGENITAL MALFORMATIONS

About four in a hundred babies are born with a congenital malformation, of which about half are serious and may threaten the life of the baby. It is a profoundly disappointing event and one that all prospective parents secretly fear. If the baby is seriously ill they also have to contend with the possibility that the baby may not survive. It is most important that the parents seek and get the maximum factual advice regarding their baby's problem as soon as possible. The nights will be long enough without needless fears from not knowing what is going on, or not knowing what his prospects are, or what surgery is necessary, and when it should be done. There are a number of special advice and support groups for many of the more common malformations,

---

I once had a patient who had bilateral cleft lip and palate. He was looked after and bottle-fed (the only way with the cleft palate), and he grew and thrived. At twelve weeks he was operated on and had his lip repaired. Soon after, mother brought him in for a check-up. She was in mild grief, missing the little baby she had been loving and looking after for three months.

LOSING A LITTLE, LOSING IT ALL

such as cleft palates, Down's Syndrome, or spina bifida, who can provide a lot of information as well as empathy and support.

Once the facts have been assimilated, the task of adjustment can begin. The parents need to see beyond the baby's problem to the little person beneath. The single malformation often throws the whole baby out of focus – for a few days the parents can see only the cleft palate. The process of grieving can slow down the acceptance of the baby and make the task of planning the future even harder.

Inevitably, the baby as a special and unique personality will emerge. The bonds form as strongly as ever, and the incredible resilience of human nature reveals itself.

LOSING A BABY

Words cannot describe the pain of the loss of a baby. A stillbirth is just as traumatic, a baby whom you have never met face to face, but know intimately.

After the baby has gone, there are so few memories to help to validate his life and make it seem more real, so the following steps are important. Try, if possible, to get photographs of the baby, to hold his image for the future. Try to get some physical contact with your baby, even after death. Within every bereaved parent there is a 'cuddle that must come out' and it is important to hold him and to say goodbye, even if, at the time, this just seems to make it hurt more. Lastly, arrange a funeral, just like you would for any other member of the family. This, too, underlines that the baby was a real person, loved and accepted by the family.

Dealing with friends

Remember, also, your poor friends. Some of them have no idea how to talk to you about your tragedy. They want to comfort you but they don't know how to start. They don't know whether to mention the baby or to avoid the subject altogether.

They may delay phoning you while they try to figure it out. Suddenly weeks have passed and they are ashamed it's been so long and it becomes even more difficult for them to call. It's hard but you may have to call them. Tell them about the baby and say that it's all right for them to talk to you about him – and not to mind if you cry when they do. They will be glad you have made it easier for them and they in turn will make it easier for you with their love and support. Other people, with the best will in the world, will say the wrong thing. Remember they are doing their best and try to ignore their clumsiness.

A life changed

No-one emerges from this experience unchanged. For some, marital relationships end, broken by the stress, while for others their marriage becomes even stronger. But for everyone, life is changed. Many parents will say that the baby they lost has taught them more about life than those babies who remained. The poignancy of death taught them more about compassion, thoughtfulness and respect for life. As we regard birth with wonder and awe,

No-one emerges from losing a baby unchanged. For some, relationships end, while for others the marriage becomes stronger

75

LOSING A LITTLE, LOSING IT ALL

mixed with joy and thankfulness, so death is the other side of that same coin, equally full of wonder and awe, but mixed with loss and finality.

It is the juxtaposition of these two staggering events that makes the loss of a newborn so difficult to assimilate.

A time for adjustment

The adjustment to the loss of a baby takes several months to years and unfortunately it gets worse before it gets better. Most parents feel that they are coping far less well after a few weeks than they did immediately following the birth, as their body and mind gradually stop protecting them from feeling the full force of the loss. They may exhibit weird thoughts and behaviours, such as the desire to search for the baby or the need to protect the baby's grave from weather. All these feelings are an adjustment and part of recovery. It is a mistake to take tranquillisers or other drugs to blunt the pain. When the drugs are stopped, the pain returns and while it remains denied it will affect other parts of life and relationships.

Eventually it has to be faced. When it is, the parents will experience intense mood swings. The so-called 'pangs' of grief will plunge them into misery and sadness. These pangs usually continue to be painful but as the months go by they will occur less often. Though nothing can decrease the pain of loss, the best help is talking to each other or to someone who cares and understands. Loving relationships can be made or broken in such crises. As time passes, the parents usually find that they suffer pangs at different times and the depressed one doesn't wish to disturb the coping one with his or her sadness. Communication slows down and the couple can drift apart.

Do not protect your partner from your feelings. You are in this together. As time goes on, you will realise that the human mind has great healing capacities far beyond anything you can imagine. The deep physical pain of your loss diminishes and the memory of your baby becomes a precious part of your past, remembered with love but without hurt. A soft ache which is the sad price some have to pay to try and achieve the joys of parenthood.

Then perhaps it is time to think of another pregnancy.

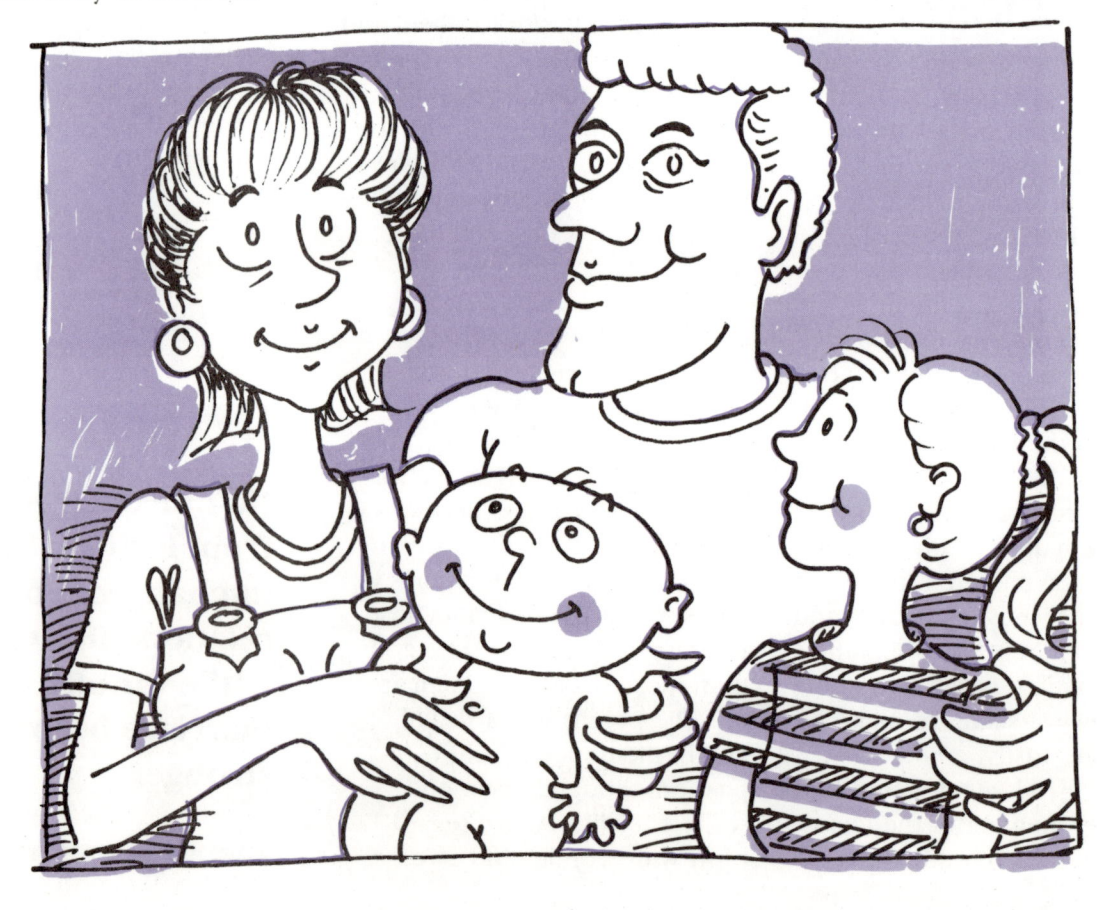

CONCLUSION

With children, as with our own life, every age has its special joys as well as those aspects we would prefer to forget. It is tempting to consider every stage our babies go through as merely preparation for the next phase of development.

Suddenly they look you in the eye and say 'goodbye' – and we wonder where their childhood went. Their childhood happened while we were waiting for them not to do that, to be a bit more mature, and not get in our way so much. It happened when they screamed all night with earache, when they ran their tricycle into the furniture and when they refused to go to bed and stay there.

Our babies are our immortality, right here and now. They are also the best personal growth experience available. Anybody who wants to tread a spiritual pathway that will hold up a mirror to the person he or she truly is, need search no further than having a baby. There is no better teacher anywhere. You can be anyone you like to your friends – compassionate, patient and sensible – but your little ones will see through the facade and show you who you really are. Like no-one else, your baby can push your secret, psychic buttons.

Parenthood is an essential part of existence, for those who wish to grow and for those who would rather avoid it.

Don't miss the opportunity or the experience.

I wish you joy and enough sleep.

Howard Chilton

The author wishes to thank Professor Jagdish Gupta for his always wise counsel and Maureen Haines who typed the manuscript.

GLOSSARY

Ammonia acrid smelling, skin irritating chemical produced by bacterial action (usually from the stool) acting on the urine.
Analgesic painkiller.
Carobel extract of carob bean similar in effect to arrowroot for thickening milk.
Cartilage white elastic substance attached to joint-bone surfaces and other parts of the skeleton.
Cleft palate defect in formation of the palate leaving a fissure in its surface.
Coagulation blood clotting.
Colostrum the first milk secreted by the breast, rich in antibodies and protein but poor in volume and calories.
Congenital present at and existing from the time of birth.
Malformation defective formation of body tissues.
Conjunctivitis inflammation of membrane lining the eyelids and covering the eyeball.
Contraindication indication against a particular treatment.
Dextrostix or **BM sticks** bedside method of measuring sugar level in blood.
Distension swelling.
Down's Syndrome specific congenital disorder affecting all body tissues caused by genetic accident.
Eczema reaction of skin with itching, redness and scaling.
Engorged excessively full.
Excision remove surgically.
Excoriation superficial loss of area of skin.
Fontanelle membrane covered space at junction of bones of skull.
Gastroenteritis infection of the bowel, characterised by vomiting and/or diarrhoea, caused by bacteria or viruses.
Granulation soft rounded mass of healing tissue.
Haemorrhage bleeding.
Heartburn pain caused by action of stomach acid on inflamed oesophagus.
Homoeopathy system of alternative medicine that treats disease conditions by giving the body tiny quantities of substances that produce similar symptoms to the disease.
Hydrocortisone naturally occurring hormone, one of whose effects is to reduce inflammation.
Lactose sugar of milk.
Leboyer French obstetrician who developed and publicised a mode of delivery that embodied a quiet, dimly lit environment to minimise psychological trauma to the baby.
Maltogen a dried extract of malt sugars fortified with vitamin B1.
Maxolon or **Bethanecol** drugs which act on the valve mechanisms of the stomach and oesophagus.
Meconium dark green mucusy material in the intestine of the fetus.
Mucus slimy secretion from mucous membrane.
Neurological disorder disease state relating to the brain or nerves.
Nystatin or **Mycostatin** antibiotic working against the fungus candida (thrush).
Ophthalmologist eye surgeon.
Oxytocin hormone secreted by the pituitary which stimulates contraction of the uterus.
Pertussis whooping cough.
Phototherapy treatment of jaundice using light to breakdown the bilirubin in the skin.
Pigmentation deposit of colouring matter within the skin.
Posset regurgitating burp.
Projectile vomiting vomiting whereby stomach contents are thrown a distance.
Pustules small white pimples of infection.
Sunkicks outmoded and potentially dangerous exposure of baby to the sun for short periods.
Saline solution of common salt in water with the same salt concentration as body tissue. To make up: dissolve one level teaspoonful of salt in one pint of water (two level teaspoons in one litre).
Sorbolene a bland white emulsifying cream.
Spasm sudden involuntary muscle contraction.
Spina Bifida congenital defect of the spinal cord and/or spinal column at the lower end of the spine.
Tibia main leg bone below the knee.
Ultrasound medical imaging technique using sound waves instead of X-rays.
Urea end product of the body's protein metabolism.

INDEX

Abdomen 23
Air travel 63
Alcohol 46
Allergies 59
Ammonia 78
Amniotic fluid 5
Analgesics 46, 78
Antibiotics 46
Anticonvulsives 46
Antidepressants 46
Antihistamines 46, 66
Antihypertensives 46
Anus 24
Anxiety 71
Apgar score 17
Apnoea 68
Arteries 23
Aspirin 46
Atopicism 59
Baby lotions 59
Back 24
Barrier cream 58-59
Bathing 25, 58-59, 73
Behaviour changes 54
Bereavement *see* Death; Grief
Bilirubin 38
Birth 4-6
Birthmarks 18-19
Blood
    clotting 16
    in stool 67
    in urine 33, 67
    test 27
Blue turns 30
Bonding
    fathers 13
    mothers 9-11
Bones
    hip 24, 26-27
    skull 21
Bottle-feeding 13, 47-49, 62
Bow legs 19, 24
Bowel action 61-62
    see also Stool
Brain damage 27
Breast enlargement, baby's 21
Breastfeeding 40-51
    and jaundice 39
    and vitamin K 7
    postnatal contractions 8
    premature babies 29
Breathing
    difficulty 67
    first 5-7
    rate 17, 18, 67
    sleep 56
Bromide 46
Burping 50-51
Buttocks, excoriated 58-59
Caesarean section 5
Cancer drugs 46
Candida albicans 60
Caput 21
Cars 62-63
Cephalhaematoma 21
Chest
    breast enlargement 21
    rattles 32

Chin 19
Cigarettes 46
Circumcision 14-16
Cleaning
    ears 25
    genital area 25
    umbilicus 37
    see also Bathing
Cleft palate 74, 75, 78
Clicky hips 26
Clothing 35-36
Coagulation 16, 78
Codeine 46
Colds 32, 66
Colic 70-73
Colostrum 41, 43-44, 78
Colour 17, 18, 19
    blue 30
    yellow (jaundice) 16, 18, 38-39, 67
Congenital 78
    dislocation of the hip 26-27
    immune deficient disease 64
    malformation 74-75
Conjunctivitis 30, 78
Constipation 62
Contact rash 58
Contraceptives, oral 46
Contractions
    during labour 4
    postnatal 8
    when feeding 43
Convulsions 67
Cortisone 46
Cot death 68-69
Coughs 66-67
Cradle cap 59
Crying 61, 70-73
Cystic fibrosis 27
Death 75-76
    cot 68-69
Decongestants 32, 66
Dehydration 46
Delivery 4-5
    examination after 17-24
    Leboyer method 10-11, 78
Demand feeding 41, 49, 51
Depression, post-natal 34-35
Developmental timetable 57
Diabetes drugs 46
Diarrhoea 67
Diphtheria 65
Dislocation of the hip 26-27
Double jointedness 26
Down's Syndrome 75, 78
Driving 62-63
Drugs in breast milk 46
Dry skin 33
Dummies 37, 73
Ears
    cleaning 25
    infection 66
Eczema 59, 78
Electronic monitoring 68
Ergot 46
Erythema, toxic 32-33
Examinations, medical 17-24
Excoriation 78
    buttocks 58-59

Eye contact 71
Eyes 21
    conjunctivitis 78
    sticky 24, 30-31
    swollen 19
    see also Sight
Face 18
    lumps 19, 36
Fat necrosis 36
Fathers 12-13, 69
Feeding 24, 25
    first two days 36
    refusal 67
    see also Bottle-feeding; Breastfeeding
Feet 19, 24
Fetus 5
Fevers 35-36, 66, 67, 68
Fits 67
Fontanelle 19, 20, 78
Foot reflex 23
Forceps marks 19, 20
Foreskin 14-16, 25
Formula milk 47-49
Fourth-day blues 34-35
Friends 55, 75
Fungal diseases 60
Galant reflex 23
Gastro-oesophageal reflux 60
Gastroenteritis 40, 45, 49, 62, 78
Genitals 19, 23-24
    circumcision 14-16
    cleaning 25
    discharge 33
Glucose 46
Gold salts 46
Granulation 78
Grasp reflex 23, 57
Grief 29-30, 75
Guthrie test 27
Haemorrhage 78
    disease of the newborn 7
Hair, body 19
Hand 19, 23
Harness for hip dislocation 27
Head 19, 20-21, 24
Health Centre Nurse 25
Hearing 22
Heart 23, 24
    rate 17
Heartburn 71, 78
Hepatitis B 65
Hernia, umbilical 23, 37
Heroin 46
Hiccups 33
Hips 24
    dislocation 26-27
Home, return to 54-55
Homoeopathy 78
    immunisation 65
Housework 54, 69
Hydrocortisone cream 58, 59, 78
Hypoglycaemic agents 46
Illness 30-33, 35-39, 58-62, 66-74
Imitation 11-12
Immune deficient disease 64
Immunisation 64-65
    natural 40, 45
    small babies 29

79

INDEX

Indomethacin 46
Infa Care 59
Ingrowing toenails 19, 31-32
Injection of vitamin K 7-8
Inoculation *see* Immunisation
Intercom 69
Intubation 6-7
Iodides 46
Jaundice 16, 18, 38-39, 67
Kidneys 23
Labour 4-5
Lactogogues 44-45
Lactose 78
    intolerance 50
Lanolin 58
Lanugo 19
Laxatives 46
Leboyer deliveries 10-11, 78
Legs 19, 24
Let-down reflex 41, 43
Listlessness 67
Lithium 46
Liver 16, 23, 38
Love 9, 11, 69
Lumps 19, 36
Lungs 5-6
Malformation 74-75, 78
Measles 65
Meatal ulceration 15
Meconium 6-7, 78
Menstruation in newborn 33
Metabolism errors 27
Metaclopramide 44
Microwave ovens 49
Middle ear infections 66
Midwife 41
Migraine drugs 46
Milia 19-20
Milk
    breast 41-45
    formula 47-49
    vitamin K 7-8
Moisturising 59
Mongolian spots 19
Moro reflex 23, 57
Mothercraft hospital 73
Mouth 21
    thrush 60
Mucus 78
    eyes 30-31
    nose 32
    vagina 24, 34
    vomited 30
Mumps 65
Muscle tone 17, 23
Nappies 25
Nappy rash 15, 58-59
Nasal drops 32
Nervous system 22-23
Neurological disorder 64, 78
Nicotine 46
Night feeds 41
Nipples
    baby's 19
    feeding position 40-43
    sore 45
Nose, blocked 66
Nystatin 60, 78
Only child 55

Oral thrush 60
Over-stimulation 71
Oxygen 6
Oxytocin 78
Pain, labour 4
Pallor 67
Paracetamol 46, 66
Pavlik harness 27
Penis 14-16, 25
Pertussis 64-65, 78
Petroleum jelly 59
Phenobarbitone 46
Phenylbutazone 46
Phenytoin 46
Phimosis 14-15
Phototherapy 38, 78
Pine-tar solution 25, 59
Polio 65
Port-wine stains 19
Postnatal contractions 8
Postural talipes 24
Prednisone 46
Premature babies 28-29
Primitive reflexes 22-23, 57
Projectile vomiting 51, 78
Questions to ask hospital staff 24-25, 25
Radioisotopes 46
Rashes 19, 25, 58-59
    milia 19-20
    toxic erythema 32-33
Reflex response 17, 22-23, 57
Reflux 60-61, 71
Relaxation baths 73
Reponsiveness 11-12
Respiration *see* Breathing
Respiratory tract infections 40, 66
Rheumatism drugs 46
Rooting reflex 23, 41
Sabin vaccination 65
Saline solution 78
Sedatives 73
Sex hormones, artificial 46
Sexual activity after birth 69
Siblings 54-55
Sickness *see* Illness
Sight 11-12, 21, 22
Skin 18-20, 58-60
    dry 33
    see also Rashes
Skull bones 21
Sleep 56, 68-69
Small babies 28-29
Smell, sense of 11
Smiling 57
Smoking 46
Snuffles 32
Soap 25
Sorbolene 59, 78
Spasm 78
Special care nurseries 29-30
Spina bifida 75, 78
Spine 24
Spleen 23
Squint 21
Startle reflex 23, 57
Stepping reflex 23
Sticky eyes 24, 30-31
Stillbirth 75

Stool
    blood in 67
    frothy 50
    loose and greenish 39
    normal 61-62
    prenatal (meconium) 6-7, 78
    watery 62
Stork-bites 18-19
Strawberry marks 19
Stress 71-72
Suctioning 6-7
Sun 36, 59-60, 78
Suppositories 62
Swaddling 72-73
Sweat glands 59
Swelling in the skull 21
Taste, sense of 11
Tear duct, blocked 30-31
Temperature 35-36, 66, 67, 68
Tension 71
Testes 23-24
Tetanus 65
Tetracycline 46
Thermometer 66
Thrush 58, 60
Thumb-sucking 37
Thyroid 27
    drugs 46
Toenails, ingrowing 19, 31-32
Toxic erythema 32-33
Tranquillisers 46
Travel 62-63
Triple antigen vaccination 64-65
Twins 51
Ulcers in the urethra 15
Ultrasound 27, 78
Umbilicus 23, 24, 25
    cleaning 37
    hernia 37
    inflammation 67
Underweight babies 28-29
Urate 33
Urea 78
Urinary tract infection 16
Urine
    frequency 25
    red-stained 33, 67
    stream 34
Uterine contractions *see* Contractions
Vaccination *see* Immunisation
Vagina 24
    cleaning 25
    discharge 33
Vernix 19
Viral infections 66
Vision 11-12, 21, 22
Visitors 55
Vitamin D 60
Vitamin K 7-8
Vomiting 25, 51, 60-61, 67, 78
    mucus 30
Vulva 24
    cleaning 25
Walking reflex 23
Water feeds 46
Weight loss 36
Whooping cough 64-65, 78
X-ray of the hip 27
Yellowing (jaundice) 16, 18, 38-39, 67